The Road to
TOLERANCE

The Road to
TOLERANCE

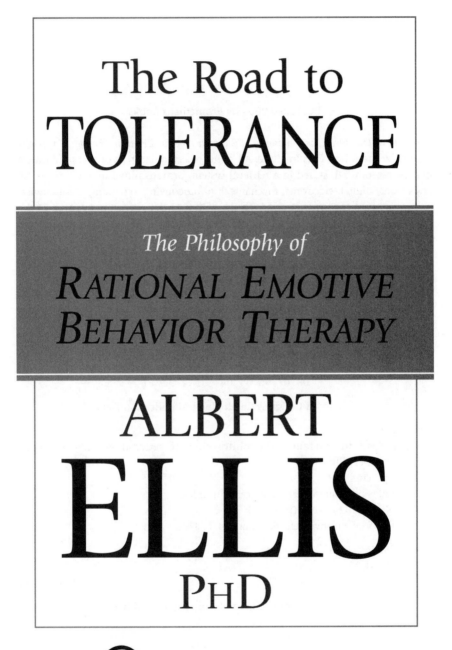

The Philosophy of

*RATIONAL EMOTIVE
BEHAVIOR THERAPY*

ALBERT
ELLIS
PhD

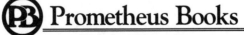 **Prometheus Books**

59 John Glenn Drive
Amherst, New York 14228-2197

Published 2004 by Prometheus Books

Inquiries should be addressed to
Prometheus Books
59 John Glenn Drive
Amherst, New York 14228–2197
VOICE: 716–691–0133, ext. 207
FAX: 716–564–2711
WWW.PROMETHEUSBOOKS.COM

08 07 06 05 04   5 4 3 2 1

Library of Congress Cataloging-in-Publication Data

Ellis, Albert.
    The road to tolerance: the philosophy of rational emotive behavior therapy / Albert Ellis.
        p. cm.
    Includes bibliographical references and index.
    ISBN 1–59102–237–1 (pbk. : alk. paper)
    1. Rational emotive behavior therapy. I. Title.

RC489.R3E467 2004
616.89'14—dc22

2004011158

Printed in the United States of America on acid-free paper

To my dear friend and assistant, Debbie Joffe, who greatly helped in innumerable respects to get the material for this book in order. Her assistance, as usual, was invaluable.

Contents

Acknowledgments

Many thanks for the constructive criticism of Emmett Velten, Kevin Everett FitzMaurice, and Debbie Joffe, who helped to make this book more accurate and readable but who, of course, are not responsible for its views. Thanks as well to Tim Runion, who did some beautiful word processing on the manuscript.

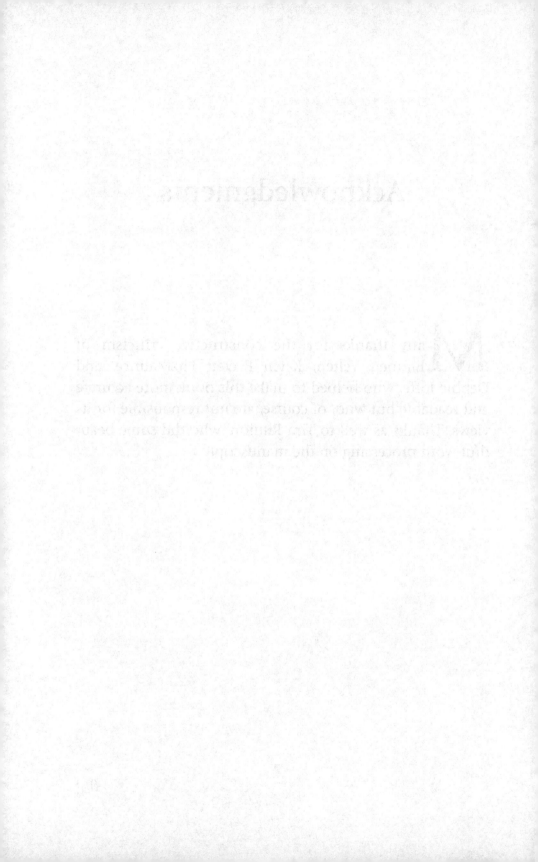

Preface

I have written or edited many books on Rational Emotive Behavior Therapy (REBT)—over seventy-five of them. Why one more? Mainly because my other books present its theory and practice to psychotherapists and counselors to use with their clients and students—but also because readers can learn the fundamentals of REBT and use them with their personal problems.

This book is somewhat different. To be sure, it again explains to professionals and those seeking personal help some of the main aspects of REBT, but it goes beyond that. I began formulating this pioneering form of therapy and counseling in 1953, when I abandoned my practice and teaching of psychoanalysis because I found it to be seriously misinformed about how and why people disturb themselves and what to do about changing with therapy. I realized, as few therapists did at that time, that people are importantly affected by their early and present environment. They are constructivists who not only *get* emotionally upset by their family members and other significant people but *also* have powerful tendencies, both innate and acquired, to construct the sabotaging of their mental and physical health. Fortunately, however, when people destructively deal with themselves and create neurotic behaviors, they also have the power to reconstruct their lives and to significantly improve. It is nice if they dig up the childhood and adolescent influences of the past, but even without doing so, they have amazing propensities for reconstructing the present and the future—that is, if they acknowledge their own disturbability and work at correcting it.

Since, as I say later in this book, philosophy was my hobby from the age of fifteen onward, I knew that some unusual philosophers had discovered and used constructivist teachings for many centuries—especially starting in the ancient Asian, Greek, and Roman eras. I therefore began to use some of their teachings to help myself with my emotional problems and physical handicaps. I give the details of this self-help practice in my companion book, *Rational Emotive Behavior Therapy: It Works for Me—It Can Work for You*, which I recommend that you read along with the present book.

I naturally used my borrowings from notable constructivist philosophers—from Confucius and Gautama Buddha to Bertrand Russell and John Dewey—in doing psychotherapy. But not enough! From 1943 to 1953, I was hardly a devoted or thorough psychoanalyst, but I was too hooked on some of its main principles to abandon them for more constructivist and existential views.

In 1953, however, after I had been a professional therapist for ten years, I made a radical break and became a severe critic of past-oriented analytic procedures, I began to develop REBT, the first major system of therapy that not only stresses the profound interaction of people's thinking, feeling, and behaving but also consciously and directly uses many cognitive, many emotive, and many behavioral techniques with virtually all clients. About a decade after I started to actively practice and teach REBT in January 1955, other cognitive behaviorists—such as Aaron Beck and Donald Meichenbaum—started to use Cognitive Behavior Therapy (CBT). Now it is one of the most widely used therapies in the world.

I am, of course, enthusiastic about REBT and CBT becoming so popular and giving rise to hundreds of empirically based outcome studies that indicate that they work with many different clients who suffer from mild neurosis, from severe personality disorders, and even from some psychotic behavior. Fine! But for many years I have realized that REBT is not only a therapeutic system but also has *general* applications to philosophy, religion, spirituality, politics, economics, and social life. It will not, of course, solve—or even aid—all human problems and totally revise our frequently destructive living. It is hardly a social cure-all!

Importantly, however, REBT has something to say about some of the central correlates or causes of human destructiveness, disorganization, and terrors that have always afflicted our lives—and still do. The more I practice therapy, the more I conclude that much personal and social evil stems from several related philosophies that have been—and still are—ubiquitous in practically all parts of the world. These are intolerance, bigotry, absolutism, rigidity,

and fanaticism. There are few, if any, emotional disturbances in which these extreme attitudes do not play an
important part. To help remove disturbance, we had better
reduce these all-too-human tendencies. That is what I and
other REBT practitioners spend much of our time trying to
do. We by no means completely succeed, but I think we
have made some real progress.

Therapeutic progress, however, considerably helps social
progress, but not completely. Along with therapy, more reor-
ganization and construction of world philosophies is, I
hope, to be accomplished. The tolerant, flexible, open-
minded views that REBT teaches individually bothered
clients have, I firmly believe, crucial implications for our
social scene. Let us recognize that!

REBT's therapeutic outlook can most probably be use-
fully applied to general social life. I have seen this over the
years and have written books, recorded cassettes, and given
workshops and lectures that promulgate REBT's therapeutic
philosophy to many social issues. This book reviews some
of these presentations and shows how they are relevant to
general human problems. It specifically includes applications of REBT teachings to philosophy, religion, spirituality,
and some social-political arenas. Its main message, again, is
that if the REBT therapeutic philosophy can be taught in
families, in the schools, in community life, in organizations,
and elsewhere to people all over the world, much less harm
and much greater good is likely to result. That means
teaching tolerance, open-mindedness, and lack of bigotry
and rigidity to all possible people. Quite a goal! Let me

hope that my speculations on philosophy, religion, spirituality, and social life will continue to help individuals with emotional difficulties—and also influence people in general to work for the betterment of the world.

1

Philosophic Foundations of Rational Emotive Behavior Therapy (REBT)

A s I noted in my prior volume on coping with my various disabilities, I was, I thought, something of a philosophic realist from the age of fifteen onward. I looked, presumably, straight at "reality," assessed its effectiveness for productive and happy living, showed how it was seriously limited in these respects, and recommended rather radical styles by which people could improve it.

I think I began thinking in this "revolutionary" way as I began seriously reading novels, plays, and do-good materials when I was eleven or twelve, especially the writings of H. G. Wells, Bertrand Russell, and a host of other do-gooders. Without too many qualms, I radically asserted to my friends and in my personal writings what *I* thought should be done with and to this world. Pronto. Directly. Definitely. Without considering too much that the consequences might sometimes be a little grim. Not many heads chopped off. Maybe a little trouble if my views were implemented. But always, of course, for ultimate human good.

Why so? First, I could clearly *see* how bad things were economically, politically, educatively, and otherwise. If they were, they had to be improved. *Had* to be. Yes. I "knew" the "right way," and (somehow) I had to bring it about. Why? Well, wrong was *wrong,* was hurting people, and was cruel, stupid, and, damn it, *wrong.* Entirely wrong? No, not exactly. But intolerably wrong. Harmful. Cruel. Unfair. Prejudiced. No sense to it.

How wrong? Even at this young age, I figured out that *really* wrong meant *needlessly* wrong: that is, it could be avoided, but practically nobody took the pains to avoid it. Of course, all humans were quite fallible. They *had* to make many errors and harm themselves and others thereby. But *unthinking, careless, thoughtless* errors? No! *Reasonable* errors—but still carelessly and sloppily made. People should—meaning, *must*—use their heads to figure out obvious harmful social errors, and quickly, determinedly push their asses to correct, or at least *try* to correct them. Otherwise, I think I thought, they *deserved* to keep suffering from their obvious blunders.

Albert, the young moralist, was I! Not that I personally had to correct people's wrongdoings by revealing them and making people change. But I certainly could be of great help and absolutely *should* be. Or else? I was really a lousy shirker. An irresponsible clod!

I summarized some of my negative views on philosophy on November 30, 1930, when I had recently reached the age of seventeen. As you can see, I was distinctly critical—but not utterly dogmatic:

On Philosophy

November 29, 1930

I have just started to read philosophy in earnest and at the present time I can say that I believe that most of the philosophy of the so-called classical philosophers from Socrates to Spencer is highly artificial and foolish. Imagine a man actually trying to prove the existence of God by reasoning and really believing in his own gibberish! Philosophers all seem to be too much influenced by religion. Besides this, their language is so complicated that it takes a genius to decipher it. Someday I shall write constructive criticism of these philosophers in language which everyone can understand. However, I may be wrong. Remember that this is only my first impression of philosophy.

A little later, I partially endorsed Couéism and its kind of mental healing. But with this caveat:

After delving into various literature on mental healing, I find the different sects all agree on a few points, such as that a physical ill can be cured mentally. This can be done by faith in one thing or another and a leader is very often necessary to aid one in getting this faith. The only mental science which I have come across which tries to explain this phenomenon scientifically is the theory of hypnotic suggestion or Couéism.

For that matter, Couéism seems to be the only logical mental science healing that there is. However, it must be admitted that no matter how unethical and preposterous the other sects, such as Christian Science, are, they certainly do obtain many beneficial results. This is due to the ignorance of their followers, but in this case ignorance is bliss.

I do not see how any person who really thinks can believe in nine-tenths of the mental healing sects—that is, really believe in their basic doctrines. However, I should advise anyone to try to believe somewhat in this foolishness, if just for the results obtained.

On my part, I believe that mental healing can be affected specifically through faith in YOURSELF not in any fates or gods. This process, unfortunately, seems to be more difficult than believing in others. However, I certainly would not advise anyone to reject modern medicine entirely in resorting to mental healing. I also advise all ailing believers and possibly nonbelievers to try some kind of mental healing.

As you can see, I stayed with faith in *oneself* and not in a higher power or in a deified hypnotist.

At the same time, I abjured perfectionism, as you can see from this excerpt from my philosophical diary in my eighteenth year:

The men and women in this world are not adapted for being perfect humans. In fact, there is not one of them, I state, who is anywhere near being really perfect.

One of the great problems to be overcome in order to have a perfect race is the problem of moods and situations. When men are in one mood they advocate something and in another mood they combat it. At one time a man will curse those people who are making noise in a theater; at another time he will make the noise himself and call anybody who tells him to keep quiet a killjoy. Then again, when a man is poor he curses the rich; when he is rich he forgets that he was once poor and cheats the poor. A freshman vows he will never bother other freshmen later, but when he becomes a sophomore he does his best to make life miserable for other freshmen. There is not anybody in this world who has not advocated one thing only to do another thing later which is against his first principle but more advantageous to him for the moment. How, then, can we ever hope to attain perfection when the very best of us are fickle in our theories?

Once again, I was far from being an extremist. In fact, I courted open-mindedness and moderation when I became a psychotherapist in 1943, as indicated by this paper that I published in 1999, when I was already a well-known therapist:

How I Manage to Be a Rational Emotive Behavior Therapist

How the hell do I leave my work at the office and stubbornly refuse to take my clients home with me? By doing the same thing with myself that I advise for the therapists I supervise at our training Institute. As you might slightly suspect, most of them are pretty nutty. No, not because they are therapists but because they are human.

For many years now I have had the quaint idea that all humans—yes, the whole six billion of them on this planet—are out of their fucking minds. No, not because I extrapolate from my clients—who are admittedly neurotic.

I also have closely observed my friends and relatives—who usually pretend to be sensible and sane. But you, having a number of friends and relatives of your own, of course know how batty they are! Or haven't you noticed?

Now I have another quaint idea—that I, too, am human—and therefore reasonably screwy. Moreover, having figured out a marvelous theory of human disturbance—which I now call Rational Emotive Behavior Therapy (REBT)—I take the unprejudiced view that it most probably applies to me, too. So I apply it.

I assume—as the principles of REBT of course brilliantly posit—that if and when I am out of my goddamned head, I foolishly make myself dogmatically *musturbate* about my goals and desires instead of merely strongly *preferring* to fulfill them. I do this as a person, as a friend, as a relative—and even as a therapist. Like other people, including the screwballs I therapize and supervise, I often construct and create—not to mention also imbibe and adopt from my not-too-rational culture—three neurotic commands and insistences:

1. I (ego) *absolutely must* be an outstanding therapist, *must* incredibly help practically all my clients, and *must* be totally adored by them—and by all my colleagues, relatives, friends, and countrymen and countrywomen as well—for being so astoundingly great! If I don't prodigiously excel, as again I *must*, I am a turd for acting turdily and I'd better go back to being a beachcomber.
2. My clients *completely must* heed everything I say, *must* love me dearly, *must always* work their asses off to help

themselves improve, and must spread the word of my miracle cures to everyone they meet. If they don't react to my therapy as they utterly *must*, they deserve to stay miserable forever—damn their stubborn hides!

3. The conditions that prevail in therapy—as well as in my general life—*unquestionably must* be totally easy, comfortable, and enjoyable! If they are not and if therapy includes any hassles, troubles, or lack of enormous rewards, it's *awful* and *horrible*! I *can't stand* it! I might as well quit and win ten million dollars in the lottery or marry a rich partner to take care of me!

Being a fallible human and having extraordinarily little power to be a perfect therapist, to induce all my clients to kiss my ass in Macy's window, and to make every single therapy session 110 percent hassle free, I have for the last forty-six years used the principles and practice of Rational Emotive Behavior Therapy (REBT) to forcefully dispute my irrational beliefs—such as the musturbatory horseshit just described—until I take it out of my head and heart and (hopefully!) stick it up my behind. Why should I insanely keep following it when I try so hard in my office to help my clients become aware of their own irrationalities and work hard to reduce them? What do you think I am—stupid?

Shall I be more specific about how I leave my work at the office? Indeed I shall. Actually, I paradoxically *don't* leave my therapy at the office. I first use it at the office itself—on *me*, I mean, and not just on my poor benighted clients. I then take it with me wherever I go: at home, at social affairs, on my trips to give talks and workshops, and when I write on planes, trains, or wherever else I can wield a pen or rattle away on a typewriter.

At all these places and in all these situations, I often make myself quite aware of my absolutistic shoulds, oughts, musts, and demands and actively and forcefully lambaste them with a number of cognitive, emotive, and behavioral methods that I constantly practice by showing my REBT clients how to use them. Employing these active-directive methods on myself, I consistently—though still imperfectly—come up with the following profound core anti-musturbatory philosophies:

1. There is no damned—or undamned—reason why I *absolutely must* be an outstanding therapist, colleague, socialite or anything else! That would be lovely and perhaps beneficial. But if few or none of my clients, supervisees, and other people approve of me and follow my teachings, that's TFB—too fucking bad! I am determined to always give myself unconditional self-acceptance (USA) *whether or not* I perform well and *whether or not* I am loved and approved.

2. My clients, supervisees, and associates never *have to* listen to me, heed my teachings, or work hard to improve themselves as I would *like* them to do. They have the right, as fallible humans, to wrongly ignore and frustrate me. It is highly unfortunate, but never *awful* and *unbearable*, for them to foolishly resist me. TS: Tough shit! That's the way they behave right now—and that's the way they *should* behave. Because, alas, they *do*! In my opinion they often *act*

badly, but they never, never, never are *bad people*! They are often *talented* at resisting my noble efforts to help them. As, again, they rightly now *should* be!

3. The conditions that often prevail in therapy don't *have to be* always easy, comfortable, and enjoyable. In fact, they often aren't. Unfortunate! Inconvenient! But not the end of the world. Just a royal pain in the ass! Now how can I do my best to improve them—or unwhiningly *accept* what I can't change? What's my alternative? More silly whining!

Do I steadily use these REBT core philosophies either in or outside of the office? No—inside *and* outside. I, still a fallible human, often bother myself while I am doing therapy—and when I am away from it. But not for long! Bullshit is bullshit—whether it be my clients' or my own. So I use the same anti-hokum with them and with myself. Even if *they* foolishly refuse to accept it, I am not exactly that stupid! Obviously not!

I can also point out that my antiextremist views have been consistent and have been applied to religion, politics, and self-helping over the years as well as to rigid REBT. A few years ago, in a paper I wrote for the American Psychological Association Convention in Chicago and later published in the professional journal *Psychotherapy*, I again emphasized antiextremism in my philosophy and practice of REBT:

The main lessons I have learned from practicing individual and group therapy with many thousands of clients for the past fifty years include the following seven:

1. Practically all clients are remarkably different, even when they have similar diagnoses and are treated with the same form of therapy. They react differently to events of their lives, to selecting a form of therapy, to how they work at the therapy they select, and to the therapist(s) with whom they work. At one time they react to therapy in one way, and at another time, quite differently.

2. Practically all neurotic clients—though not necessarily borderline and psychotic ones—are in some ways remarkably similar in the manner in which they disturb themselves. Almost all of them have innate tendencies to take their strong desires and preferences (which they learn and which they also have biological predispositions to construct) and to escalate them into unrealistic, illogical, absolutist demands and to thereby disturb themselves when these rigid imperatives are not fulfilled. They often dogmatically construct and rigidly persist in upholding these absolutist commands—especially (a) "I *absolutely must* perform well and be approved by significant others!" (b) "Significant others *absolutely must* treat me kindly and fairly!" and (c) "The world *absolutely must* provide me with easily achieved pleasures and few real difficulties!" What percentage of the world's five billion people frequently hold these neuroticizing ideas and thereby fairly often engage in self- and social-defeating behaviors? Approximately 100 %! Fortunately, however, almost all of them are born and reared with constructivist, self-actualizing tenden-

cies that, especially with good therapy, enable them to think about their crooked thinking, and to think about thinking about their thinking, and thereby to minimize their neurotic reactions.

3. Practically all therapists are remarkably different and individualistic in following the form of therapy that they claim to practice. They often work quite at odds from the theories they say they hold and from the techniques they say they use.

4. All forms of psychotherapy work to some degree with some of the clients some of the time. These range from "scientific" and "rational" forms of therapy to highly "irrational" methods.

5. "Irrational" and "unscientific" therapies often help people to overcome their presenting symptoms, and sometimes to make an important personality change, for a number of reasons: (a) Clients come to therapy strongly believing in these methods or acquire a powerful belief in them during treatment. (b) "Irrational" therapies are persuasively presented by therapists who believe in them, sometimes with the use of effective persuasive materials. (c) "Irrational" therapies wittingly or unwittingly include powerful "sensible" elements along with their "outlandish" ones. For example, Alcoholics Anonymous irrationally holds that problem drinkers are unable to stop drinking on their own and *need* a spiritual force or Higher Power to help them do so. But it also includes many sensible ways of showing AA members how to change their stinking thinking.

6. Not all forms of therapy work equally well with most clients most of the time. Some modes work significantly better with certain types of clients and/or with those who have specific symptoms. However, some therapeutic methods, if used by competent therapists, work better with more clients more of the time than do some of the other therapies. These effective therapies tend to include a number of cognitive, emotive, and behavioral methods rather than focusing on one main technique.

7. Most therapies help many clients to *feel better* when they come for therapy but only a few therapies help them to *get better*. Getting better includes: (a) Reducing one's presenting symptoms. (b) Acknowledging and reducing other related and unrelated symptoms. (c) Becoming less disturb*able*, so that when unfortunate life events occur (or one makes them occur), one has significantly less of a tendency to seriously upset oneself about them. (d) Remembering, if one reverts or lapses to feeling disturbed again, that certain therapeutic methods were originally helpful and working at using these methods again.

Although I agree with Arnold Lazarus and Hans Strupp that most clients make modest rather than profound changes in successful psychotherapy, some of them actually *get better* in the sense of becoming significantly less disturbed *and* less disturb*able*. That is the goal for which I usually urge my own clients to strive. Of course, they don't *have* to achieve it—and my insisting or their insisting that they *must* do so is damned crazy. But I have a strong preference for them to feel better *and* get better; and I usually push my ass to push their asses to achieve this great result!

As a therapist, I was also philosophical in general. Soon after I enthusiastically started to teach—yes, teach—my clients to use REBT with their own problems, not to mention the problems of others with whom they related, I also started to amalgamate it with my views on philosophy, religion, politics, and—though I hardly recognized it at that time—spirituality and purposiveness. I suppose that, to a considerable degree, everyone does—that is, everyone attempts to "prove" that her or his basic views on "important" matters go with each other and "make good sense."

I was helped to do considerable "consistencizing" of my views in several conversations with Lyle Stuart, Paul Krassner, and Robert Anton Wilson—all of whom agreed with much of my outlook but also asked some relevant questions about it. These questions and my answers to them were included in a widely distributed interview that Paul and Bob wrote up for the March 1960 issue of Paul's thoroughly iconoclastic *Realist*. While I did not expect this interview to range from REBT to practically everything under the sun, it did so—and became the semiofficial word on REBT and its ramifications.

Although I might well tone down some of its views, I still hold most of them today and think that the interview with Paul and Bob is an early manifestation of REBT philosophy and is still largely accurate. Here is my "Impolite Interview" of 1960 and its slight 1983 revisions. Over four decades later it is still going strong!

Questions Posed by Robert Anton Wilson and Paul Krassner

Q. How would you explain the difference between rational emotive behavior therapy (REBT) and psychoanalysis?

A. There are many significant differences between these two systems of psychotherapy. In fact, the techniques most used in classical psychoanalysis tend to be least used in REBT.

In psychoanalysis, the most important procedures involve free association, dream interpretation, analysis of the client's past history in minute detail, and analysis of the transference relationship between the client and the analyst. The assumption is that if one gets clients to understand how they became disturbed, somehow their newly found insight will—rather magically, I would say—clear everything up and they will marvelously change.

Another assumption is that if clients work out various difficulties in their relationship with the analyst, they will thereby learn to work out similar difficulties in their relationships with others.

When I was practicing classical analysis, and later when I practiced psychoanalytically oriented psychotherapy, I found that some of these assumptions simply do not work; and many other practicing therapists have independently made the same discovery.

I found, for example, that you can give clients loads of insight and they still often do not improve. You can show them exactly how they got to be emotionally disturbed in the first place and again they don't significantly improve their feelings or their behavior.

And you can work on and work out all kinds of involved love-hate relationships between the client and the analyst and, perversely enough, many clients still do not generalize their analytic transference teachings and sagely apply them to their outside relationships.

Because I found, after several years of my practicing classical analysis and analytically oriented therapy, that many of the Freudian and neo-Freudian assumptions simply do not work, I gradually evolved the system of Rational Emotive Behavior Therapy (REBT) which I now employ and which is used by thousands of other therapists throughout the world.

In the course of REBT, the focus is largely on what is happening to clients during the present, and particularly on what they tell themselves about what is happening. Their past history is briefly considered, and some important aspects of it may be related to present behavior. But this is only a small part of the therapy.

The main thing is to show clients that any so-called feeling or emotion that they now experience is accompanied—and usually explicitly or implicitly preceded by—ideas, cognitions, evaluations, beliefs, self-statements, and/or images that they fairly strongly hold. Frequently (but not *always!*), people's underlying (and occasionally deeply unconscious) beliefs or cognitions are not symbolic, vague, or hazy but mainly consist of simple declarative—or exclamatory!—sentences or verbal self-statements. But these beliefs or evaluations can also be held in other ways and may largely consist of meanings, assumptions, and philosophies of which people are not fully aware, and which may occasionally be deeply unconscious. The theory of REBT holds that, whether they are aware of it or not, people mainly react to their own expectations or philosophies and not only or mainly to the things that happen to them.

In rational emotive behavior psychotherapy, a considerable portion of the time—which on the whole tends to be much briefer than the time spent in psychoanalytic therapy—is spent in showing clients what are their own internalized beliefs, how irrational these are when they lead to disturbed feelings, and how they can be clearly observed, parsed, challenged, questioned, and changed.

REBT is the main brand of therapy, therefore, that most directly and forcibly induces people not merely to see and understand their own basic assumptions and self-assertions but ruthlessly to question and challenge their assumptions—to beat them over their goddamn heads—until clients no longer self-defeatingly hold them.

Q. You've written about "the A-B-C of rational psycho-therapy"—namely: that "A" is what people perceive, "B" is what they believe about what they perceive, and "C" is their reactions not to "A" but to "A" plus "B".

Now, then, isn't it possible that after a while, part "B" becomes eliminated and that—more or less like a Pavlovian-type reaction—a person will react to "A" directly with "C", leaving out "B", the internalized sentence?

A. Do you mean when the person has disturbed reactions?

Q. When he's disturbed?

A. When emotionally disturbed, people seem to automatically react to stimuli at "A"—for example, someone trying to insult them—with a "conditioned" reaction, "C" (such as feeling anxious or angry).

Actually, however, no such simple "conditioning" is going on, and I do not think that Pavlov himself thought that it was. He developed a theory about what he called the "secondary signaling reaction," which implies that even in the case of his famous "conditioned" dogs, more is going on than at first meets the eye.

Thus, the dog initially salivates when he sees and smells the food. Then, when a bell is rung just before the food is placed before him, he becomes "conditioned" to respond to the bell and salivates as soon as he hears it, even before the food is placed before him. This looks, on the surface, like automatic "conditioning"—a kind of psychological magic.

Actually, however, the dog is signaling himself something when he learns to connect the bell with the food, and he is therefore—at which I call point "B"—telling himself, in his own way, something about the bell and its connection with the food. After this self-signaling takes place—even though it may occur within a fraction of a second after he perceives the food—he salivates. It may look like it is the sound of the bell alone—at point "A"— which causes his salivation, but actually it is his self-signaling, or his interpretation of the bell and its connection with the food, and this self-signaling takes place at point "B".

Q. **And is this fact—that the "B" is still there—is this**

what allows you to be successful in REBT? If the "B" were gone, wouldn't you have as much difficulty as a psychoanalyst who finds what the original trauma was, but still doesn't do the client much good?

A. Yes, if people still, at the time they came for therapy, did not give themselves a hard time at point "B", still did not catastrophize about or childishly rebel against what was happening to them at point "A", REBT would not be able to help them very much. Because that is what we do in Rational Emotive Behavior Therapy: question clients' unrealistic and irrational interpretations and conclusions at point "B".

In addition, in REBT we not only teach clients to recognize their self-defeating beliefs at point "B", and to actively challenge them, but we encourage them to *act* against these beliefs—for example, to do some of the things they falsely believe would destroy them. We urge clients to get off their asses into direct action, so that they thereby, ideologically and behaviorally, decondition their needless fears.

Q. Could you give a specific example of how that works?

A. Certainly. In the case of a man who is terribly afraid, let us say, to ride in subways, a rational therapist would first get him to see that his fears consist of some beliefs such as "I will suffocate if I ride in subways," or "If I go into the subway I may feel faint, and people will stare at me and pity me and that will be awful." He would then be shown how to challenge and contradict his own beliefs: to ask himself "Why would it be so terrible if I feel faint in the subway and people stare at me?" or "How will I really suffocate in a subway station?"

In addition to this challenging of his own inner verbalizations, the client would be induced, as part of his therapeutic "homework," actually to take some subway rides, and, in the course of these rides, to observe his specific feelings and the ideas behind these feelings.

If necessary, he would be encouraged and persuaded to go on subway rides time after time, until he became most clear as to what he was "bugging" himself about on such rides and until he became habituated to doing what he had previously been afraid to do. His irrational "B" would thereby be contradicted both in theory and in practice.

Q. Isn't there a basic flash, sort of, which represents a person's set of assumptions at point "B"—a basic flash of what you say is an internalized sentence?

A. Yes, sort of. People have a basic belief system, or system of values, which they consciously or unconsciously strongly and emotionally believe. And this belief system instantaneously flashes, if you want to use that term, into their heads every time they contemplate a certain feared activity.

Thus, in the illustration just given, the man who fears subway rides may have the basic philosophy, or set of beliefs, that it is terrible if people stare at him in a pitying manner. And this philosophy, this series of fundamental *assumptions* that he holds at point "B", induces him, in any given case where he contemplates taking a subway ride, to "flash" to himself, "Oh, no! I couldn't do that!"—which is a logical deduction from his illogical or irrational premise—namely, that it is terrible if people stare at him in a pitying manner.

It is this irrational premise we would clearly bring to awareness and persistently and strongly (emotionally) challenge.

Q. What do you think of Conditioned Reflex Therapy?

A. On theoretical grounds, it has some points in its favor, since Andrew Salter, who originated this form of therapy, induces clients to go out and act, for example, extrovertedly even though they may feel introverted. If he can actually get them to do this, they help propagandize themselves against their fears of introversion—since action is one of the very best forms of self-propagandization—and thus tend to overcome their fears.

Unfortunately, however, most clients will *not* go out and act against their fears unless, coexterminously with asking them to do so, the therapist also concretely shows them how to depropagandize themselves ideologically by perceiving, challenging, and contradicting their own self-suggested nonsense. Conditioned Reflex Therapy does not properly emphasize this ideological self-analysis and restructuring of the client's philosophy; hence, its results tend to be limited.

Q. Would you say the same limitation applies to the "positive thinking" panacea?

A. Definitely, yes. Many people think that rational therapy is closely related to Emile Coué's autosuggestion or

Norman Vincent Peale's positive thinking, but it is actually just the reverse of these techniques in many ways. It is true that clients become emotionally disturbed largely because of their own negative thinking or autosuggestion, and that is why they sometimes snap out of their depressions and anxieties quite quickly—if temporarily—when they are induced to do some kind of positive thinking or autosuggestion.

But accentuating the positive is itself a false system of belief, since there is no scientific truth to the statements that "Day by day in every way I'm getting better and better"—which was Coué's creed—or that "Because God loves you, you need have no fear of anybody or anything," which appears to be Norman Vincent Peale's latter-day version of autosuggestion.

In fact, this kind of Pollyannaism can be as pernicious as the negative claptrap which clients tell themselves to bring about neurotic conditions.

In REBT we do not merely stress positive thinking or autosuggestion, but a thoroughgoing revealing and uprooting of the negative nonsense which clients endlessly repeat. Scientifically, this negative nonsense can be analyzed and refuted, since it is largely definitional and has no empirical evidence behind it.

As I tell my clients in the vernacular, their continued repeated negative thoughts are invariably bullshit, and if I can get them objectively to look at this crap they are telling themselves (for example, "I can't possibly ride in the subway," or "How awful it would be if so-and-so did not like me")—then they have no need for any grandiose views that God is on their side or that everything will happen for the best.

Another way of putting this is to say that no matter how often a woman repeats, "Every day in every way I'm getting better and better," or "Jesus loves me, therefore I am saved," if she keeps saying to herself much louder and more often, "I'm really a shit; I'm no fucking good; I'll never possibly get better," all the positive thinking in the world is not going to help her. Unless she is forcefully led to challenge and undermine her own negative thinking, as in effective cognitive psychotherapy, she is still a gone goose.

Q. Incidentally, you may recall, a couple of issues back in the *Realist*—this was in regard to my satirical thing on the birth control primer and Bob (Wilson's) piece about the reaction to it—the Tolerant Pagan in his column said something to the effect that you can express any thought without being boorish. Why—by his standards—do you deliberately make yourself out to be a boor?

A. Why should I live up to his, or for that matter any other individual's, standards? My own standard is that certain modes of expression, including the use of many of the famous or infamous four-letter words, are unusually appropriate, understandable, and effective under certain conditions and at these times they can be unhesitatingly used. Words such as *fuck* and *shit* are most incisive and expressive when properly employed.

Take, for example, the campaign which I have been waging, with remarkable lack of success, for many years, in favor of the proper usage of the word *fuck*. My premise is that sexual intercourse, copulation, fucking, or whatever you wish to call it, is normally, under almost all circumstances, a damned good thing. Therefore, we had better not use it in a negative, condemnatory manner. Instead of denouncing someone by calling him "a fucking bastard" we can say, of course, that he is "an unfucking villain" (since bastard, too, is not necessarily a negative state and should not only be used pejoratively).

Q. Isn't the apparently inconsistent use of the word *fuck* **due to the fact that it actually has two meanings. One, it means intercourse. The other, it means screw— you know, like in business—"I fucked him."**

A. You're right. But since the word *screw* has the same two meanings and since screwing is (in my unjaundiced view) equally enjoyable to fucking, I would want the usage to be "I unscrewed him," when we mean that I outwitted him or gave him a rough time.

Q. How about the famous Army saying, "Fuck all of them but six and save them for pallbearers." There, fuck means kill.

A. Yes, and it is wrongly used. It could be "Unfuck all of them but six." Lots of times these words are used correctly, as when you say, "I had a fucking good time." That's quite accurate, since fucking, as I said before, is a good thing, and a good thing leads to a good time. But by the same token you can say "I had an unfucking bad time."

Q. I can see this, you know?—In the subways, two or

three centuries from now: "Unfuck you!" on the Hunt's Tomato posters, say.

A. Why not? It's fuckingly more logical that way, isn't it?

Q. Speaking of logical—at what age can you begin to teach a child to control negative emotions in a logical, rational way?

A. It is not a matter of teaching children how to *control* their emotions. It is rather a matter of teaching people philosophies of living different from the negative philosophies which now produce disordered emotions, and, through teaching these different philosophies, to help them *change* rather than to *control* their feelings.

As far as children are concerned, I recently saw an eight-year-old boy and decided to try some rational therapeutic techniques with him, just to see how effective they might be. This child, a bright but very disturbed boy, stuttered quite badly and was not only upset because of the stuttering but because his friends and relatives kept teasing him about it.

I was able to show the boy that it really wasn't too important if others teased him and that he need not—at point "B"—upset himself about their teasing by telling himself how awful it was. I quoted him the same nursery rhyme that I often quote my adult clients—Sticks and stones/Will break your bones/But names will never hurt you—and I told him that he need not be hurt by the teasing of others and that he could stop upsetting himself if he recognized that these others had their own problems and that their words didn't really matter very much.

It was amazing some of the things that this boy said back to me after the third session I had with him—showing how he had really understood what I said and that he was beginning to see that no, he need not be upset by the words and gestures of others, and that it really *didn't* matter that much when he was teased.

By the end of the fourth session, he was not only much less disturbed about being teased, but actually was stuttering a lot less and he has continued to make remarkable improvement, even though I have seen him only occasionally. Apparently, bright eight-year-olds can also benefit from REBT—sometimes. In fact, more than their more difficult and prejudiced elders.

I've also tried rational methods with young adolescents in several instances and I have frequently been able to show them that, whether they like it or not, their parents have problems, that they don't have to take these parents too seriously (particularly when the parents are highly negative toward the children), and that they don't have to get upset just because the parents are disturbed.

Here again, I show these adolescents that it is not only what happens to them at point "A" (their parents' negativism) that really depresses or destroys them but also their own catastrophizing and awfulizing beliefs: "They *must* not be that unfair to me!" "They have *no right* to act that undesirable way!"

Q. Would you call this a form of preventive therapy?

A. Yes, that is why I, Dr. Janet L. Wolfe, and my other REBT associates have founded the Albert Ellis Institute in New York City, with branches in many parts of the world. The

Institute runs a clinic for individual and group psychotherapy clients, conducts workshops, seminars, and lectures for the public, and trains REBT therapists. But it also
does research in Rational Emotive Education (REE), teaches
teachers how to use REE in classroom situations, and pub-
lishes and distributes printed and audio-visual materials on
REE.

In educational centers that are REE-oriented, children
are taught rational philosophies and coping statements,
are instructed in the ABCs of REBT, and are given regular
group therapy sessions where they can learn to detect and
dispute their own Irrational Beliefs (IBs). My hypothesis is
that if, in addition to receiving conventional education,
children attended an REBT-oriented school from kinder-
garten to the eighth grade, they would develop much
better methods of self-understanding and self-help than
other children and would become significantly less emotionally disturbed adolescents and adults.

**Q. I think that, in many ways, rational therapy is sim-
ilar to General Semantics. A lot of what you tell your
clients to do—to determine the irrational interpretations which they communicate to themselves—is what
Alfred Korzybski told people to do when he said they
should extensionalize what's actually happening in
terms of actual physical events rather than high abstrac-
tions about what they feel about their situations. Do
you think your system is close to that of General
Semantics?**

A. I think that in theory we're very close. I had very little
knowledge of the General Semantics people until I started

using Rational Emotive Behavior Therapy. Then I was informed of what they were doing and began to subscribe to their journal, *Etc.*, and I find that their views are much to my liking.

I have read Wendell Johnson and other leading General Semanticists and I haven't as yet found any of them who has thought out and applied a thoroughgoing system of psychotherapy based on their own principles. In fact, I would say that REBT is pretty much the answer to much of General Semantics theory—which their group still largely *theorizes* about and which we actually *practice*.

Q. Well, Wendell Johnson is just one of the General Semanticists. There are others with different approaches.

A. Yes, I am sure there are. And much of what I do is implicit in the ideas of Korzybski and some of the other General Semanticists. But whereas they are somewhat general, I really do get at my clients' specific irrational, overgeneralized, and vague thinking. I encourage them to look at, to parse their own internalized sentences, and, what is more important, to change them for more efficient, more logical internalized beliefs.

When I speak about REBT to a group of the General Semantics people, they are very cordial on the whole—much more cordial, indeed, than a group of my fellow psychologists often are. The psychologists are sometimes hostile to my theories because they tend to have highly biased, unscientific Freudian views, and many of them could benefit considerably from General Semantics teachings.

Q. There are Humanists, too, at the meetings of the General Semantics society which you address, aren't there?

A. Yes, the Humanists are one of the main groups which overlap to some extent with the General Semanticists. The Existentialists, too, or at least some of them, overlap with this kind of thinking and with major parts of my own views. They see, for example, that it is clearly people's philosophy of life, and not just the things that happen to them, which importantly affect their personality development.

But Existentialist therapists, while clearly revealing to and analyzing patients' worldviews, and showing how they relate to their emotional disturbances, are often namby-pamby when it comes to helping them *change* these views. Like the classical psychoanalysts, they apparently believe in the magic power of insight—while REBT practitioners believe in *using* understanding along with emotional and behavioral methods.

Existentialist therapists usually forbear from attacking and undermining patients' childish, irrational assumptions, and in this respect they are relatively ineffective in helping them.

Q. Doesn't the Adlerian school of therapy also closely overlap with your therapy?

A. Yes. Adler, too, pointed out, and in fact was one of the very first to point out, that it is individuals' mode of life, or irrational goals, which activate disturbance. And the Adlerians are more vigorous than most other therapists in examining the clients' poor life plans.

But many Adlerians still tend to be more analytical than persuasive in their approach, and they emphasize social interest rather than enlightened self-interest as a worthwhile goal. REBT stresses both enlightened self-interest balanced with social interest as goals (as indicated in my book with Dr. Robert A. Harper, *A Guide to Rational Living,* and my book with Dr. Irving Becker, *A Guide to Personal Happiness*).

Q. Dr. Russell Meyers, the neurosurgeon, has a theory he calls attitudinal sets. He says that people respond to stimuli with complete attitudinal sets, by which he means they have a sentence—one of your internalized sentences—and they respond in a physical reaction to which the whole organism responds, according to a pattern of attitudinal sets that they've learned as they've grown up.

You don't emphasize the bodily aspects as much as he does, I gather. You're just after the verbalization that people make inside themselves?

A. Yes, I mainly emphasize people's seeing and attacking their own philosophies. But I also admit that bodily reactions, or motor behavior patterns, do not *automatically* disappear when one faces and changes the internalized sentences, or philosophies of living, which cause and sustain these reactions. One still has to force oneself into physical counteractivity, as well as perform emotional-experiential exercises.

Thus, if one tends to become nauseated because one is telling oneself that a certain kind of food is disgusting, one will not automatically begin to like this food if one merely depropagandizes oneself in regard to its "disgusting" quality. One had better *also* on several occasions, *while* attacking one's own negative internalized sentences about the disgustingness of the food, force oneself to try this "disgusting" food. As a result of both processes, self-depropagandization and motor counteractivity, one finally ceases to be nauseated.

In REBT, in other words, the emphasis is not only on counterattacking one's own self-verbalized, attitudinal sets, but there is also a strong emphasis on changing motor behavior as well. REBT often encourages people to try new physical and bodily paths and first to make themselves uncomfortable, to emotionally tolerate this discomfort, and then perhaps to become comfortable and enjoying.

Q. A psychiatrist told me once that the reason the Freudian method often doesn't work is because no abreaction occurs—the client remembers but doesn't relive the experience—and he said that this type of emotional abreaction has to go along with remembering.

A. I disagree. I think that abreaction is often a waste of time in therapy because merely reliving an original traumatic event may help clients see better, get more significant insight into their problems, but it still will not necessarily help them to attack their basic irrational philosophies and dysfunctional feelings that are mainly causing disturbance.

Remember that it never was, in the first place, an original traumatic experience that made people disturbed but their *attitude toward* this experience—at what I call point "B". Thus, if someone makes a public laughingstock of you when you are a child, it is not the experience itself but your idea that it is horrible to be laughed at, which really upsets you at this time, and much of your so-called traumatic experience really includes this emotionally held idea.

Therefore, abreacting this experience many years later will hardly help you to change this idea, unless in the course of reliving the experience you also see that it is *not* horrible to be laughed at, and that neither originally nor in the present *need* you upset yourself about this experience.

Moreover, many clients, when they relive past experiences, get so much satisfaction out of their abreacting— have such a dramatically good time in the process—that they actually get distracted from their real problem, which is to change their *still existing*, irrational philosophies and feelings.

In a few cases, clients not only abreact but, in the course of doing so, somehow say to themselves, "Jesus Christ, now I see clearly how I upset myself about things in the past. But I don't have to be similarly upset *now* about the same kind of thing. Who the hell *wants* to go on acting in this emotionally childish way? I had damned well better stop this crap."

Under *these* circumstances, clients may well get better—*not* because of abreaction but because of what they tell themselves about abreacting experiences and because of how they change the ideas (with or without the therapist's help) that originally produced much of their trauma.

Q. I'd like to get your opinions on some other schools of therapy. What do you think of the Jungians?

A. On theoretical grounds, I would be opposed to much of Jung's writings, since he was quite mystical, believed in a racial unconscious, and often recommended religious observance to his clients. On the other hand, in his book on *The Practice of Psychotherapy*, he stated that his own technique was a combination of the Freudian and Adlerian methods, and I get the impression that he was actually more Adlerian than Freudian when working with clients.

My main criticism of the Jungians is that when they do what I would call effective psychotherapy—which some of them certainly do—their practice does not really stem from their theory and they are being pragmatic rather than theoretical. Similarly, many so-called Freudians do effective therapy, but they invariably do so because, consciously or unconsciously, they are ignoring Freud's views on technique and are empirically discovering for themselves what clients find helpful.

Whenever I address a group of psychotherapists, someone in the audience invariably arises to state that what I call REBT is pretty much what he does in his own practice. Yes, I reply, but I do it on the basis of my *theory* while you do what you are doing on the basis of your own common sense and in spite of the therapeutic theory in which you say you believe.

To get back to the Jungians, Carl Jung is to be given

due credit for emphasizing the idea of individuation. And where Jungians attempt to get their clients to be true individuals in their own rights, and not to give too much of a damn what others think of them and their individual tastes and preferences—there, I and the Jungians compatibly overlap.

Q. What do you think of Wilhelm Reich?

A. Do you mean as a sexual theorist or as a therapist?

Q. Well, Reich felt that if you had a so-called perfect orgasm, you could meet any problem—you could withstand any difficulty that arose during the day.

A. This particular Reichian theory, I am afraid, consists of some of the worst bullshit ever written, since no orgasm, perfect or otherwise, is really going to solve an individual's major personality difficulties. In fact, as I have said on several occasions, so-called sex problems are almost invariably the result rather than the cause of basic problems of thinking and emoting—of personality disorders.

Let me hasten to add, however, that Reich wrote an excellent book, called *The Sexual Revolution*, which is very liberal and enlightened and contains some good material. Unfortunately, he also wrote an incredibly bad book, *The Function of the Orgasm*, which has highly perfectionist notions of what a "normal" orgasm should be, and which has helped thousands of males and females to be more sexually and generally disturbed than they otherwise would be.

Reich's original idea of the individual's acquiring a character armor, and consequently also developing muscular and visceral tensions and armorings, has a certain measure of truth in it. He took this idea, however, to ridiculous extremes and ended up by believing that if therapists massage and manipulate clients' bodily zones, they will break up clients' armoring and thereby loosen neurotic traits. More bullshit, I am afraid.

What the Reichians do not seem to understand is that if one massages and masturbates clients, which is essentially what Reichian therapists will do if they strictly adhere to their own theory—even though one's physical manipulations are largely worthless—one is unwittingly depropagandizing them of some of their sexual puritanism while doing this poking and massaging.

Thus, if John Jones irrationally thinks that sexual participation is a wicked business, and his Reichian therapist (particularly if she is a female therapist) keeps pleasingly poking him often enough, Jones is quite likely to start saying to himself: "Well, what do you know! Sex can't be so wicked after all." And he may actually lose some of his inhibitions and unhinge some of his character armoring.

The question is, however: Is it really the Reichian pokings that are helping the patient or is it the new ideas that these pokings are giving him?

Q. But don't you do much of the same thing in REBT, though without the aspect of positive transference which the Reichians or Freudians may employ? In other words, don't you induce your clients to get their sex outside of therapy, instead of during the therapeutic process?

A. Right. Quite honestly and openly, I frequently (though not always) will work with sexually inhibited individuals and will frankly encourage them to try masturbating or having intercourse—outside the therapeutic relationship. And I help them have these relationships not because they love or hate *me*, but because it is better for them to engage in such relationships, and because I am able to uproot their negative, puritanical ideas, so that they then have the freedom to enjoy themselves sexually.

Reichians and other therapists often do the same thing as I do—but quite indirectly and inefficiently, I would say, and with a certain amount of attached hypocrisy. And hypocrisy, or lying to oneself, I need hardly remind you, is one of the main cores of emotional disturbance.

Q. I can just see a client of yours saying, in the after-glow, "Dr. Ellis would be so proud of me for doing this."

A. Yes, this actually happens at times—but in spite of, and not because of, what I do—because I am not at all interested in clients doing anything for *me*, but only for *themselves*, and I teach them that when they do things to please me, they still haven't solved their own problems.

Once, for example, I saw a man who had had five years of analytic therapy before I saw him and who wasn't getting far with his current analyst because when he went out with women he never had the guts to put his arm around them, let alone make any other sexual passes. He came to me, after his analyst had thrown in the sponge, and said: "What shall I do?"

"Very simple," I replied. "You make a regular date with the woman you have been interested in for some time and take her to a movie. In the movie, you sit next to her—say, on her right. Now, if necessary, you take your left hand in your right and you push—yes, push—it over to her."

Said he: "You really mean that?"

"Absolutely. You'd better stop your shilly-shallying and make some physical move toward her."

"Okay," he rather reluctantly said. "I'll try."

So he called up his friend, took her to a movie, and sat next to her for a half hour, debating as to whether or not he was going to make a move toward her.

Q. There was more drama going on in the audience than on the screen.

A. Yes, there certainly was. Finally, he said to himself— just as you predicted in your question—"Hell, I can't go face Dr. Ellis if I don't make some move here." So he literally did what I had told him to do: took his left hand in his right hand and pushed it over to the girl. Whereupon, she practically grabbed his hand off, and from that time on they got along physically as well as mentally.

Often, my clients tell me that when they are trying to do something that they are afraid of, and are having great difficulty doing it, they literally hear my voice saying, forcibly repeating: "Now what are you afraid of? What the fuck difference does it really make if you get rejected? What's *really* going to happen to you that's so terrible?" and so on. And they then go and do the things they've been terribly frightened of doing.

But this is only the beginning. Unless I can get these same clients, a little later on, to do things because *they* want to do them, and not because they want to please me or anyone else, and unless I can get them to heed their *own* internalized sentences, instead of responding to those I have given them, they will still go on believing the same hogwash that originally caused them to be emotionally disturbed, and they will not really get better.

Q. To go on with some of the other schools of therapy—what do you think of Erich Fromm?

A. Until recently, I have always been an enthusiastic reader of Fromm, since he has said some most intelligent things and has, for the most part, a similar attitude to loving and being loved that I have worked out in my own theorizing. In his latest works, however, particularly *The Art of Loving*, he goes a little too far and tends to help make people guilty if they're not among the very loving.

Fromm especially exaggerates because he sees, truly, that intelligent human beings had best do *something* or have *some* long-range, devoted interests outside themselves, but he seems also to assume that this outside interest *must* consist of loving others. As I explain to my clients on many occasions, anyone with reasonably good brain cells is not likely to be very happy in life if he or she does not have some definite vital absorption. But absorption may mean being distinctly concerned about (a) people, or (b) things, or (c) ideas, or (d) any combination of (a), (b), or (c).

Outstanding creative artists or inventors may go

through life never caring much for other humans and may still be reasonably sane and emotionally healthy—as long as they are sufficiently devoted to whatever major field or project they enjoy.

Fromm seems to think that you must be devoted to another person to be a full person yourself, and this to me is a very narrow view. It has a grain of solid truth in it, but it's much too narrow.

Q. Well, Fromm also thinks that if you're in love with just one person, there's something wrong with you.

A. Yes. In-lovedness he considers to be, as I also do to some extent, an obsessive-compulsive attachment that can often (though not always) be disturbed. But he has no objection, nor do I, to loving another.

Q. What distinction do you make between "loving" and being "in love"—and can they be simultaneous?

A. In some respects loving and being in love are aspects of the same basic emotion, but in other respects they are almost opposites. Being in love is often little more than a genteel term for having an obsessive-compulsive fixation on someone, and this is something of a disturbance.

Being in love, however, is statistically normal, since most of us are in the state one or more times during our lives; and it is a state that has distinct advantages, in that it is highly absorbing, often pleasurable, and sometimes positively ecstatic.

In-lovedness, moreover, usually lasts for only a relatively short period of time, rarely for more than a few years, while loving may go on indefinitely.

Loving, as Erich Fromm was one of the first clearly to point out, means being interested in another human being for her own sake and from her own frame of reference. Whereas the man who is violently in love usually demands return love, and often falls madly in love as a thinly veiled excuse for being able to demand reciprocation, the loving individual is not that interested in reciprocation.

Loving, in fact, often stems from personal strength— meaning, that loving people do not really care that much whether others love them and are therefore strong enough to be truly interested in others. It is altruistic but not particularly self-sacrificing, since, at bottom, the loving individuals enjoy and like themselves and have no need to sacrifice their own major interests to win the approval of others.

Q. Would you agree or disagree with the proposition that altruism is the highest form of selfishness?

A. I would agree if by altruism you mean interest in another person that basically stems from one's own self-interest—which we often mistakenly label as "selfishness." I usually put it this way: People who are truly self-interested, who live their lives on the supposition that the ninety or so years that they have on this earth is it, and they then are going to be dead as a duck for all eternity, and who therefore try to get as much of the things they want and as little of the things they don't want during this relatively brief existence—these people are rational and sane.

As a result of their rationality, they will tend to have two corollaries to their existence:

First, they will normally avoid needlessly and deliberately harming others, since in so doing they would tend to invite recrimination and to create the kind of a world in which they themselves cannot fully flourish.

Second, they will be so unanxious and unhostile toward others that they will have little to do in life but to become vitally absorbed in some kind of major outside interests—and these interests may well include loving or being devoted to helping those who are younger or weaker or whom they find lovable.

In other words, the more one is determinedly self-interested in an intelligent and enlightened way, the more altruistic one will usually (though not always) tend to be. Self-interest, especially if it includes a dearth of overconcern about what others think of one, logically leads to sincere interest in selected other persons, things, and ideas. At bottom, it is proaltruistic.

Q. How do you feel about sexual freedom for teenagers?

A. Although, as I have stated in my books, I feel that premarital sex relations are fine for those who are sufficiently intelligent, well-informed, and emotionally mature to avoid unwanted pregnancy and venereal disease, teenagers are unfortunately often not in this category.

They frequently are uneducated, ill-informed, and emotionally immature. But I have my famous "out" for them even in these instances—namely, that if they refrain from penile-vaginal coitus, which could well lead to undesirable results, they may still quite freely engage in petting to orgasm, which is likely to have only good results.

Q. Well, if they're well-informed enough to pet to orgasm, wouldn't they also be intelligent and mature enough to use contraception?

A. Not necessarily. It is easier to teach many teenage youngsters to pet to orgasm and avoid actual intercourse than to have intercourse and always to employ proper contraceptive technique. Almost any teenager can be taught: "Do what you may sexually, with the full consent of your sex partner; but rigorously refrain from intercourse because it may well lead to pregnancy. Other than that, go enjoy yourself up to the hilt!"

Q. You mean NOT up to the hilt, right? . . . What do you think of D. H. Lawrence?

A. I am afraid that Lawrence was something of a prude! In spite of his real courage in writing works such as *Lady Chatterley's Lover*, he was a prude in his attitudes toward masturbation—which he considered essentially wrong and almost wicked—and toward the sexuality of women.

He was morbidly afraid of females and throughout several of his books, such as *Aaron's Rod* and *Women in Love*, he keeps portraying an active, aggressive woman who's out to deball her lover by keeping after him sexually, striving for her own orgastic satisfaction, and sapping his strength and vitality.

Lawrence, during a large part of his life, had very serious sex problems and had considerable feelings of inadequacy about his potency and his "masculinity."

Like so many disturbed males today, he falsely identified masculinity with his sacred penis and his ability to give a woman a simultaneous orgasm during penile-vaginal coitus. This was very sad, since Lawrence otherwise had the capacities to be a free and unanxious human being.

Q. But—judging by some of his essays, such as "Pornography and Obscenity"—wasn't Lawrence, rather than antimasturbation per se, antimasturbation when it's done as a kind of secondary thing instead of intercourse, with people getting their kicks vicariously through movies and novels rather than with an actual sex partner?

A. Perhaps so, but in the essay you cite, he did refer to "the vice of self-abuse, onanism, masturbation, call it what you will." He felt that masturbation is "exhaustive"; that it includes no sexual give and take, as intercourse does; and that "in masturbation there is nothing but loss." These are rather extreme statements.

Certainly, as I have pointed out in *Sex without Guilt*, masturbation is usually *less* satisfying than heterosexual copulation, but it is hardly exhaustive unless, like Lawrence, you are prejudiced enough to think that it is, and it endows many human lives with utterly harmless and enormous benefits that these lives otherwise would miss.

Lawrence, moreover, wrongly assumed that extrav-

aginal methods of heterosexual contact were masturba-
tory—when, of course, they include just as much give and
take, and often a lot more, than does vaginal coitus.

**Q. But would you agree that in masturbation—well,
there's no togetherness?**

A. Yes, there is no togetherness in masturbation. But
millions of people masturbate most joyfully without
any need, at that time, for togetherness, even though
they find it in other sex acts. And, unlike Lawrence's
hypothesizing, these millions frequently do not find
masturbation frustrating; quite the reverse—they find
not masturbating highly frustrating.

**Q. All right, but since we may assume that average mas-
turbators use their fantasizing powers, isn't there a
danger, especially over a prolonged period of time, that
their need to store up and refer to sexual imagery will
become a habit pattern?**

A. Why shouldn't it? We all fantasize about having an
enjoyable meal at times, and that hardly interferes with
our actual enjoyment of eating. As I have shown in *The Art
and Science of Love*, the sex lives of many married couples
are largely saved by the fact that they can fantasize all
kinds of exciting situations while having intercourse
together, while, if they relied on thinking only about each
other, they might never be as sexually competent.

Fantasy, creative imagery, or whatever you want to call
it is the very core, and the particularly *human* core, of a

good sex life. Naturally, emotionally disturbed people can abuse their fantasizing powers, but less disturbed individuals can make marvelous use of these same powers.

Q. Would you call it healthy or unhealthy when a person who has practiced sexual imagery over a long period of time in the course of masturbating finds it necessary to use this imagery to help himself obtain sexual satisfaction while actually copulating?

A. Ordinarily, I would call this use of fantasy effective and, in that sense, healthy. For we have to face the biosocial fact that many individuals do become relatively bored sexually with their mates and that they are unable to achieve full satisfaction unless they fantasize other partners during intercourse.

Females, in particular, are poor bedmates in many instances because they have trained themselves to do little or no fantasizing during sex relations. I have to teach many couples to fantasize before they become sexually adequate and gratified.

Q. What kinds of fantasies?

A. All kinds, from very loving to extremely sexualized imageries. Many women, for example, have to make up an entire love story in their heads before they become fully aroused. Thus, they daydream about meeting a man, going to dinner, having him tell them how lovely they are, going home with him, and so on and so forth—a dream-lover sort of thing.

And, without such fantasies, they may be unable to masturbate or have heterosexual intercourse. Other women have very specific sex fantasies, including those of copulating with a man other than their husband, and I often help them to overcome their guilt about having these kinds of fantasies.

Q. Wouldn't the fact that you've been married and divorced twice seem to detract from your efficiency as a marriage counselor?

A. Not necessarily. For one thing, by being married and divorced twice one may acquire first-hand experience which is not too often acquired and, through this experience, gain an understanding of certain aspects of marriage that may be very valuable in counseling.

Ultra-romantic views, for example, are likely to be dissipated by down-to-earth marital experience, and, providing one does not become bitter or cynical, a realistic view of marriage is important for a marriage counselor.

Second, through having the guts to acknowledge one's twice-made mistakes, and do something about them, one is likely to acquire self-acceptance and courage that may well serve as a good model of behavior for one's marriage counseling clients.

Third, a considerable number of people who come for marriage counseling actually have already made up their minds that they want a divorce and want to be helped through what might be called divorce counseling. Here, the counselor's personal experience with marriage and divorce may well be helpful.

For several reasons such as these, I feel that my own experience with two marriages and divorces has been exceptionally useful to me in my marriage counseling practice.

Q. What do you think of the dating system?

A. Pretty crummy, in more ways than one. Not only does it lead to much sex nonsense, with the couple trying to outwit each other instead of trying to discover a good basis for a mutual sex-love relationship, but it also is a poor way of matching individuals for love or for marriage. This is particularly true in the case of the highly intelligent and cultured person.

The average individual who is a high school graduate and is interested largely in sports, TV shows, and cheap magazine fare—may be able, just because he or she is average, to meet a few members of the other sex and to like or love one of these few. Almost by definition, the average person will have average tastes and will be relatively easy to please when it comes to choosing a sex-love partner.

Not so, however, the above-average individual—say, the person who has a high I.Q. and is interested in aesthetic-cultural pursuits. Such an individual very frequently will have to meet thirty, fifty, or a hundred members of the other sex before he or she can expect to find his or her "soul mate."

But our contemporary dating system, with its restrictions on how and where it is permissible for one to meet a member of the other sex—particularly if one is a female—makes it difficult for the above-average individual to meet the relatively large number of other-sex partners he or she had better meet if his or her selective requirements are to be met.

Q. Do you have any possible solution?

A. Possibly. First, on an individual level, above-average— or, for that matter, even average—persons in this society can be taught, largely through the methods of REBT, to ignore many of the unnecessary restrictions of our culture and to make a much wider variety of contacts than he or she would normally—or should I say abnormally?— make.

The main reason why so many young people (as well as older unmarried individuals) stick to the conventional dating mores of our society is that they are afraid *not* to do so—are afraid, in other words, of being rejected, being spurned, being looked down upon by members of the other sex to whom they might be attracted. But in the course of REBT, whether it is done on an individual or a group basis, people learn that there is nothing to be afraid of in being rejected or spurned by another—that their "hurt" or "depression" at being rejected stems from irrational ideas in their own heads, from invalidatable premises that they unthinkingly keep telling themselves.

To put this into the A-B-C terms, people who successfully undergo an REBT psychotherapeutic experience learn and come to believe that it is not, let us say, a partner rejecting them at point "A" which makes them desperately "hurt" or "depressed" at point "C". Rather, it is the nonsensical sentences that they believe at point "B", about what happened at point A. These beliefs usually take the form: "Oh, how awful, how terrible, how frightful it is that So-and-So rejected me! I can't stand her thinking so badly of me. I'll never take the horrible risks of such a rejection again!"

Q. When they can instead be saying . . . ?

A. When they can instead be saying: "It's too goddamn bad that So-and-So rejected me, and I wish to hell she hadn't, but that's the way things are. Tough! Maybe I'll try her again next week; what have I got to lose? And if she still irrevocably rejects me, tough again! I won't like it, but I can stand it. Even if ninety-nine partners reject me, there's always the hundredth."

I've now seen literally thousands of clients who were thoroughly bound by our restrictive dating system when they first came for therapy and who have now been released and are taking chances and making overtures to partners that they would never have dared to make previously. And you'd be surprised how many of them are having more than their share of success.

Q. What do you think of pornography?

A. As literature, I feel that most of it stinks. It is exceptionally badly written, trite, and boring. I hardly read any amount of it. In its own right, however, it sometimes has a place in helping to arouse individuals so that they can achieve greater sex satisfaction. This is largely because direct sexual representations are banned in our society and, as D. H. Lawrence pointed out, made secret. As I note in an essay on "Art and Sex" in the *Encyclopedia of Sexual Behavior*, pornography gets its effectiveness because it depicts acts which are against our mores, and if we really want it to lose its appeal, we had damned well better change those mores.

Q. Do you think that there is any kind of writing or graphic representation that should be banned?

A. I can't think of any. I think that it's quite legitimate for some person or group to advise, or even warn, others not to patronize certain forms of writing or pictorial art. But it's not legitimate for this person or group to enforce, by law, a ban against the works they consider sexually dangerous.

It's the question of vice versus sin. Addiction to pornography may well be a human vice in some instances, but I cannot see that it is sinful and punishable. Though I believe that some people are emotionally disturbed in their addiction to pornography—because they spend thousands of dollars in their obsession with it and neglect many other enjoyable aspects of living in the process—I think that human beings have a right to be emotionally immature.

And others have a right to advise them: "Why don't you go for help, get psychotherapy, and overcome your emotional disturbance?" Just as these others have a right to say to their gambling-addicted associates: "Why don't you go for psychological help so that you can stop squandering all your money at the racetrack?"

But I still am opposed to banning pornography. People, if they are adults and have been warned against being vice-ridden, have the right to retain their vices.

Q. What do you think of Henry Miller?

A. Henry Miller is often an unusually fine writer. In such books as *Tropic of Cancer*, *Tropic of Capricorn*, and *Black Spring* he has done exceptionally good work. In some of his later books, such as the *Rosy Crucifixion*, he goes to ridiculous lengths (such as having a character copulate with his mate in a crowded movie theater) and becomes boring and unbelievable.

Q. What religions do you think do the most harm to people's sex lives?

A. Virtually all orthodox religions—including orthodox Catholicism, Judaism, Protestantism, etc.—include specific antisexual rules that enormously influence and interfere with the sex lives of their adherents. Liberal religions, such as reformed Judaism and liberal Protestantism, seem to inflict the least sexual harm on their believers.

Q. Do you think that sexual neuroses created religions or that religions created sexual neuroses?

A. First of all, I doubt whether there is such a thing as a sexual neurosis per se, since most individuals I find with severe sexual problems have a general [neurotic] outlook, and as a part and parcel of their general neurosis they develop a so-called sexual neurosis. So let me turn your question around somewhat and ask: do I think that neuroses created religion or that religion created neuroses?

Partly, this is a matter of definition. Because if we define both in their broadest sense, I think that they are the same thing and that therefore neither created the other but both stem from the same fundamental source.

That source may be called faith unfounded on fact, human gullibility, lack of scientific thinking, an unquestioning and unchallenging attitude toward life, or a refusal to accept and live with reality when it happens to be grim.

Originally, I believe, both religion and neurosis got started because people had genuine problems—such as rainstorms, forest fires, lack of food, and difficulties of living together in groups—about which they had insufficient knowledge to solve, and not being able effectively to control these real problems they built up substitute or quasi-solutions, particularly consisting of obsessive-compulsive rituals and the blaming of self and others.

That is to say, not being able to control or solve the immense problems of storms and hunger, they dreamed up deities to whom they kowtowed and for whom they ritualistically punished themselves—so that these gods, presumably, would solve their problems for them.

And not being able to control or solve the large personal problem of how to get along well with others and still maintain their own self-respect, they dreamed up what might be called subdeities, such as compulsive personal rituals (handwashings, withdrawal from social contact), or constant status-seeking, or ingratiating conformity, or other neurotic symptoms.

Another way of putting it is to say that ancient people seemed to have the basic philosophy that if you cannot control a large area of living, such as climatic conditions or your own interpersonal relations, you had better pick on a smaller area—some ritual—that you know you can control and then assume that the control of the smaller area automatically will help you with the control of the larger one.

More specifically, you had better assume that if you make sacrifices or punish yourself in relatively *little* ways, the unkind fates will somehow magically protect you in *big* respects.

This belief is, of course, a non sequitur and has little or no evidence to support it, but if it is held strongly enough, it will lead to the (false) certainty of support—and, peculiarly, that very false certainty will temporarily help you, in many instances, feel better about the original problem.

Unfortunately, however, it will not at all help you really to *solve* the problem. Indeed, by diverting your feelings, and making you falsely believe that the problem *has* been solved, it will hinder you from ever solving it.

This, in a nutshell, is both dogmatic religion and neurosis: the establishment of a false or unprovable belief—faith unfounded on fact—which gives one the illusory sense that one has solved real life problems for which one, usually quite unwittingly and unconsciously, created the unprovable belief in the first place.

Because one (again unconsciously) really seems to believe that problems cannot be solved—and, remember, primitive man really *did* have climatic and other problems that could hardly be fully solved at the time—one develops a "solution" that pushes it out of mind and lets one somehow assume that it now is solved.

More specifically, after assuming that one *cannot* by one's own efforts control rainstorms and floods, one invents a deity who presumably *can* control these occurrences, and then one also assumes that certain self-punitive or self-sacrificing rituals (virtually all of which are annoying and work-involving pains in the ass) will help one control one's assumed god.

In regard to so-called sexual neuroses, the same kind of thing happens. After having sexual difficulties (usually because we think we are fundamentally worthless and that we will be miserable failures in our sex relations), we look around for some magic means of controlling our sexual responses and hit upon some fetish (such as having our sex partner wear high-heel shoes) or symptom (such as compulsive masturbation) and work very hard at controlling this aspect of our sex life.

We thus delude ourselves that God and fate are on our side and that we will be sexually competent, and because we believe this delusion, we often are somewhat in control of our sexuality.

At bottom, then, devout religious beliefs and neurotic beliefs are the same kind of magical means by which disturbed people "control" their world and deflect themselves from actually tackling and solving some of their basic problems.

Q. Would you say that the basis of your technique of Rational Emotive Behavior Therapy can be epitomized by developing the client's ability to say, "So what?"

A. No, not quite, but the statement that REBT partly consists of teaching clients to say and, what is more important, to *mean*, "So what?"—has some degree of truth in it.

Let me put it this way. Emotional disturbance normally consists of overconcern rather than of sensible concern for what is happening. Disturbed people seriously exaggerate the significance of something—especially, of what others may think of them, of how terrible it would be for them to fail at something, of how awful it is to feel disturbed.

It would be difficult for them to be disturbed if they were utterly realistic—that is, if they accepted unchangeable and inevitable things as they are, instead of unrealistically contending that they *should* or *must* be different from the way they are.

This does not mean, of course, that the individuals should not try to improve conditions of living. And it certainly does not mean that they should believe that everything must happen for the worse and that therefore there is no use in trying to better life situations.

For although this latter tack may seem to be a sensible "So what?" attitude at first blush, it is really a catastrophizing, "My-God-isn't-everything-positively-awful-I-had-better-completely-give-up-trying" attitude.

In other words, if you are overconcerned or awfulizing about the people and things in your life, you will either be anxious most of the time or may adopt an un-fuck-it-all, defensive so-whatness point of view. This latter kind of "So what?" attitude is precisely what REBT does *not* teach, since it is only a mask for underlying overconcern.

What we therapists *do* teach is that there is nothing for

people to be *over*anxious about, nothing to be *over*afraid of. More specifically, REBT teaches them that there are literally millions of instances where it *doesn't* make much difference what your neighbors think of you or what wheels are turning in other people's heads.

In these many instances, you can appropriately learn to say: "So what? So what if everyone doesn't love me? So what if I try something and fail at it? Will it really kill me? Will my world really end?" This is the kind of so-whatness that REBT promotes. But not lack of concern for important troubles that may occur.

Q. You're not saying, though, that people should never give vent to negative emotions—by, say, crying—are you?

A. No. There's nothing wrong with good honest sentiment, such as crying, when something has really gone wrong in your life—when a close relative, for example, has died.

Regret, sorrow, grief, irritation, annoyance, displeasure—many kinds of negative emotions, such as these, are perfectly legitimate reactions to deprivation and frustration. We don't get what we would like to get and we're sorry: If we were happy under such circumstances, it would be most inappropriate—in fact, downright crazy.

But when we convince ourselves that loss and failure absolutely *must* not exist, and when we dogmatically *command* (instead of *wish*) that they disappear, we then turn our legitimate regret and frustration into anxiety, depression, and hostility. We then needlessly *make* ourselves emotionally disturbed and dysfunctional.

That is what's wrong and what REBT opposes. It teaches people once they have illegitimately translated legitimate regret and frustration into severe anxiety and hostility, to re-translate them back into less self-defeating feelings—that is, into sorrow and annoyance.

Reason, when truly worthy of its name, does not—as is so often unreasonably assumed by its opponents—do away with human emotion. It merely enables individuals to keep their natural, legitimate feelings within practical limits and to use them for maximum enjoyment.

Reason can be effectively used as a tool to destroy exaggerated, self-defeating, highly negative emotions, but not, if it is still to remain worthy of the name *reason*, to do away with all human emotions. That wouldn't be living!

Q. Rational therapy has been compared to Zen—yet you've said that Zen is like throwing out the baby with the bathwater. We quoted this to Alan Watts and he disagreed. What's your reaction?

A. It is quite possible that in Alan Watts's personal brand of Zen, indifference to the inevitable—or contemplation of one's navel—is not taken to extremes, and that he can therefore remain vitally interested in life while still being, in a sense, totally detached.

But other devotees of Zen often not only throw out emotional pain (through their doctrine of accepting the inevitable) but leave out desire as well. Like REBTers, they not only eliminate necessity or need but they also extirpate desire or preference.

When I, personally, get to *that* point—the point of

giving up *all* my human desires—I doubt whether I shall see any good reason to live.

Still other Zen Buddhists have various mystical—and, to me, rather impractical—doctrines along with their quite sane acceptance of grim reality and of human individuality.

Thus, the noted Zen propagandist Huineng espoused the doctrine of no-mind or mindlessness. Starting from the proposition that "From the first not a thing is," he reasoned that seeing into one's self-nature is nothingness—since self-nature is "not a thing." This is as far from REBT as I can imagine any doctrine to be!

Similarly, many other Zen Buddhists, along with their valuable insights into the intrinsic existence of a human being, include mystical mumbo-jumbo and impractical rituals. Alan Watts may not be of this group, but there are apparently Zen Buddhists and Zen Buddhists.

Q. Yes—Inners and Outers. . . . What about Ayn Rand's philosophy of "objectivism?"

A. Ayn Rand's and Nathaniel Branden's objectivist views are in a few respects quite sane, rational philosophies of living. She is logically against extreme self-sacrifice—or what I call Florence Nightingalism—and I certainly agree with her. But her views of "free" capitalism are extreme and impractical.

By the same token, the "objectivist" school believes in the absolute power of human reason, and although I am rational, I am not a philosophic "rationalist" and do not believe in the absolute power of anything.

I believe, along with Hans Reichenbach, that we live in

a highly probabilistic world, where nothing seems to be absolutely certain. And REBT tries to help people to accept this kind of world and to be able to live happily in it.

More specifically, Ayn Rand seems to believe strongly in blaming human beings for their mistakes and errors and punishing them—if necessary, by death—for their wrongdoings. In rational psychotherapy, we accept mistakes and wrongdoings as unfortunate facts of life but never damn anyone for anything.

The kinds of people Ayn Rand excoriates in *Atlas Shrugged* are not, to my way of thinking, bastards, villains, sinners, or lice, even though they may often be deluded and wrong-headed. It is the job of an REBTer to show foolish people how and why they are wrong, and how they can change for the better, rather than to hate their guts and damn them for being horrible "sinners." REBT espouses unconditional self-acceptance instead of highly conditional self-acceptance that Rand fanatically fights for and also endorses unconditional other-acceptance. It may deplore what people *do* but never damns them for their *behavior*.

Q. Where do you draw the line between self-sacrifice for others and self-sacrifice for oneself? How about the sacrifices of Albert Schweitzer, for example?

A. I cannot accurately assess Schweitzer's motives, so I cannot be certain what kind of self-sacrifices he made. I can easily see, however, how an individual such as Schweitzer might aid his own sane self-interest by in some ways sacrificing himself for others.

What I am strongly opposed to, and what I meant

before by Florence Nightingalism, is the notion that unless you deliberately and consistently sacrifice yourself for others, and put their interests ahead of your own, you are a wicked, selfish individual and don't deserve to live.

In REBT we teach that sane individuals normally put themselves *first* and primarily go after what they really want out of life—while, at the same time, taking care to help others and to work for a happier world.

REBT shows people that it is usually *desirable* but not *necessary* for them to help or devote themselves to others, since in having this kind of social interest they tend (especially in an atomic age!) to create a better life for themselves. To some extent going out of your way to help others can be one of your greatest satisfactions and may lead to maximum self-efficiency and pleasure. But if you choose mainly to be self-interested and "selfish," that is your prerogative and you are hardly a worm!

Q. Are you a "Rational Fascist?"

A. No, although I fully admit that there are those who are rational fascists. But I, for one, do not believe in rational thinking as an absolute good or a certain solution to all possible problems. I admit that a rational approach to life is a value judgment rather than a scientific "fact," and that those who wish to be irrational are fully entitled to *their* value judgments.

I uphold the hypothesis that if you want a certain end in life, especially of not being anxious or hostile, I can show you how to think more rationally and thereby attain that goal. But I have no intention of *needing* or *forcing* you to be rational, even though I believe that you most probably will be better off if you did favor rationality.

If, then, you *want* to be irrational and to contend, with Spengler, Ortega y Gasset, and other thinkers, that irrationalism is a good thing, that is your prerogative. If you uphold the thesis that everyone in the world might just as well commit suicide or that we all should devote our lives to mystical mumbo-jumbo, I again will uphold your right to believe and preach this doctrine. This is your value system, and, for better or worse, you have a right to it.

Rationality is not good for all purposes, but only for specific goals. If you want to be desperately unhappy, for example, I would strongly advise you not to attempt to be rational!

But if you want—as millions of people in this world seem to want—real, consistent freedom from anxiety and hostility, from shame and blame, then I doubt whether you're ever going to be able to achieve your goal unless you definitely employ logico-rational methods of thinking.

So I don't think that I am a rational fascist in that I try to *impose* my views on others or that I dogmatically contend that they *must* be the best views. I merely say, on theoretical and clinical grounds, that I strongly believe that if you want certain ends, my system of Rational Emotive Behavior Therapy will help you achieve them. If you want certain other ends—such as anxiety, guilt, despair, hostility, and depression—it is quite probable that some non-rational technique will best serve you.

Q. Final question: Are YOU happy?

A. I think I can honestly say that I am one of the relatively few people in the United States, and perhaps in the entire world, who has not had a seriously miserable day since I created REBT in 1955.

I find it almost impossible to feel intensely depressed, hostile, or upset for more than literally a few minutes at a time. I really would have to start working myself up to be miserable. I'd have to work hard at, to practice again, disturbing myself.

Whereas I was desperately unhappy for a good part of my childhood and teens, this feeling is virtually unknown to me today. Instead, these days, I almost automatically go after self-disturbances and quickly eliminate them. Not squelch, suppress, or repress them—I mean really eliminate.

And because I have so little time and energy to expend at making myself miserable, I derive considerable pleasure, enjoyment, and sometimes sheer bliss out of my life. What more can one ask?[1]

*   *   *

A more up-to-date description of how I apply the philosophy and practices of Rational Emotive Behavior Therapy to my clients and myself is shown in this interview I had with Lara K. McGinn, PhD, for the *American Journal of Psychotherapy* as the twentieth century drew to a close:

Q. Perhaps we could start with having you summarize the tenets of Rational Emotive Behavior Therapy for readers who may not be familiar with it.

A. Well, Rational Emotive Behavior Therapy (REBT) says that all people are born [and raised] with self-defeating tendencies. When something goes against their goals, values, or desires, usually failure and rejection, they have a choice of feeling healthier emotions such as feeling sorry, disappointed, frustrated, which encourage them to go back and change the adversity they face. Or humans have a choice of making themselves terrified, panicked, depressed, self-pitying, and self-doubting.

Which emotion they choose mainly depends on their belief systems. Not just their goals and values but what they tell themselves when those goals and values are thwarted or blocked. And they have a rational set of beliefs or what we call "preferences" or self-helping beliefs, such as "I don't like what is going on; I wish it weren't so, how annoying; let's see what I can do about it." Or people very frequently pick irrational beliefs or what we call "demands," such as "because I don't like what is going on, it absolutely should not exist, it must not be! I can't stand it! It's horrible! I think I'll kill myself!"

There are only three basic demands that lead to most of what we call neurotic behavior. One is, "I must do well and be loved by people or I am no good," which leads to depression, terror, self-doubting, and feelings of inadequacy. Two, "Other people absolutely must treat me kindly, nobly, and considerately, or they are worthless, they are no good!" That creates anger, rage, wars, and genocide. Three, "Conditions under which I live in my environment must absolutely be better than they are, must give me exactly what I want, and never really deprive me! It is horrible, terrible, and awful when conditions are not the way they must be!"

REBT is more philosophical than the other therapies because it helps you change your basic outlook, philosophy and give up those musts, shoulds, oughts, and demands and merely go back to having preferences. "I would like to do well but I never have to. It would be great if you treat me kindly but you obviously don't have to." If people stick only to their preferences, they would rarely make themselves neurotic. And if people use many cognitive, emotive, and behavioral techniques which REBT shows them how to use, by working very hard against their [irrational] upbringing and their biology, they could make themselves significantly less disturbed.

So these, very briefly, are some of the main aspects of REBT, which was the first of the major cognitive behavioral therapies since I created it in 1955, and then about ten years later Aaron Beck came along and Donald Meichenbaum, and then William Glasser and others who have somewhat similar systems. But they don't emphasize the musts, the shoulds, and the oughts as much as we do. They go after irrational beliefs but they often miss the core beliefs, "I must do well, you must treat me well, and things must be easy."

Q. So could you describe some of the techniques that are used in REBT?

A. The main things in REBT are the "ABCs." You start with "G" or the goals (to do well, to get along with people, to enjoy yourself). All humans who survive have goals, values, desires, part of which again are innate and part of which are learned through your parents, your culture. "A" is Adversity or Activating events that block or thwart your goals.

"B" is what you tell yourself about "A". It's your Belief system, both your healthy, rational belief system, preferences, and goals ("I don't like 'A'; I wish it weren't so") and your unhealthy, irrational belief system, demands, oughts, musts, shoulds ("Therefore, it shouldn't exist. I know the right way, you know the wrong way, and you absolutely should follow my way!").

"C" is your emotional and behavioral Consequence, which is often your actual disturbance. Usually it is your feelings—anxiety, depression, rage—but it is also behaviors—procrastination, or compulsive thinking, or smoking.

Finally, "D" is Disputing, questioning, challenging your irrational beliefs until you change them back to preferences.

Your cognitive, emotional, and behavioral techniques consist of finding and disputing your irrational beliefs and ending up with realistic preferences. REBT includes many emotive techniques to help people feel differently because they often strongly hold on to their beliefs. If they only lightly dispute them, they get what is called "intellectual insight," they say, "it's true, I don't need your approval, I only prefer it," but underneath they are saying "I really do, I must have it." Therefore, they had better *strongly* believe, "No, I definitely do *not* need your approval, though it would be nice to have it."

Q. What about the behavioral techniques?

A. We have a whole host of behavioral techniques where we get people to do what they are afraid of, do public speaking, go for job interviews, approach members of the same or opposite sex. And we also give them reinforcements and penalties. For example, if they don't do what they are irrationally afraid to do, or if they continue smoking or drinking, etc., they may give themselves a stiff penalty such as sending $100 to a cause that they hate.

Q. How do you think REBT has changed over the years?

A. Well, originally, I thoroughly emphasized the rational side. But over the years, I have acknowledged that people very strongly hold on to their beliefs, so I created a bunch of emotive techniques like my famous "shame-attacking exercise," where people are encouraged to deliberately do something foolish in public and not feel ashamed. We have several other techniques, including some we took from the experiential and encounter therapies. And now we keep advocating, more so than ever before, behavioral techniques that are supported through research, such as in vivo exposure and desensitization and also staying in an uncomfortable position, such as with a rotten boss or in a bad marriage, until you stop upsetting yourself about it and then you decide whether or not you are going to change.

Q. What kinds of psychological problems does REBT treat?

A. All psychological problems that any other therapies treat. We often see people with psychoses, those with severe personality disorders, and those on medication as well. We seldom treat seriously retarded people, but we treat the whole range of emotional and behavior disturbances.

Q. What led you to develop the theory and therapy?

A. At first I was a pretty active-directive therapist when I got my MA degree in 1943 because I had done considerable research on sex, love and marriage, and sex therapy, which has been cognitive-behavioral since the early part of the century. But then I thought that psychoanalysis was deeper, more intensive, so I got analyzed and practiced psychoanalysis for six years. But I found that my clients were often getting worse rather than better. So, in 1953, I stopped calling myself a psychoanalyst and did a survey of the scores of therapy techniques that were popular and took the best of them. I felt that many therapies were woefully ineffective, so I formulated REBT in 1955 with the goal of making therapy more efficient. At that time there was little behavioral therapy, just Skinnerian and classical behavioral therapy, and there were lots of emotive therapies, Fritz Perls and others, but they tended to directly enhance feelings without distinguishing between unhealthy and healthy feelings.

My purpose was to make therapy more efficient and profound and to get to the basic source of human disturbance. I wanted people to work hard rationally, emotionally, and behaviorally against their tendencies to be destructive, to go back to their constructive potentialities, which they also have, and to finally lead a more self-fulfilling and happier life.

Q. What were your influences at the time?

A. My main influences were philosophical. I happened to have a hobby of philosophy since the age of fifteen. There were some cognitive influences, but I really got my main theory that people largely upset themselves from ancient philosophers, some of the Asians, but also from the Greeks and Romans.

Q. You are one of the pioneering psychotherapy developers. As such, your career has been filled with many accolades and accomplishments. When you look back, are there any disappointments in your career? Is there anything you wish you had or had not done, or perhaps done something differently?

A. Yes, lots of things. For example, I was one of the first to use so-called improper language in public, which turned some people off. I am not sure whether it does more harm than good. And lots of times I have argued with therapists, told them that they are wrong and created enemies. Perhaps if I had been more tactful . . . (*smiles*).

Another thing that never worked out is research. We founded the Albert Ellis Institute as a training institute in 1959 and we pushed for our trainees to do research. We had several directors of research. All of them have fallen down on the job and produced very little important research. We also spent thousands of dollars trying to get our therapists to do some basic research in REBT, and they've done some, but relatively little, while other people have done better in colleges and universities. And other cognitive behavioral therapists, such as Aaron Beck and Donald Meichenbaum, have done considerable research. But I regret that I was never able to induce our people to do much more basic research.

And I have done many other things that I regret but I never upset myself about those things. They're just regrets, sorrows, disappointments, frustrations. I made mistakes, I am a fallible human who has made mistakes. Too bad. But I never put myself down for making these errors.

Q. What do you personally consider to be the greatest satisfactions of your career?

A. Well, I have gotten many awards. I have received the major awards from the American Psychological Association, the American Counseling Association, and the Association for the Advancement of Behavior Therapy. I am probably the only one who received all three. So that is nice. And I have given workshops and trained therapists all over the world. So I have done many things that I enjoy and that I think have been helpful. Plus, I probably see more clients than any therapist in the world.

Q. How many clients do you see?

A. Well, every week I have four groups, so that is thirty-two people right there. I also see fifty other people individually. And I have been doing this since the 1950s. I know few therapists who have seen more clients than I have over the years. I also do workshops every Friday. Since 1965, I have interviewed people in public every Friday night that I am in New York. I have a regular live session with two different people and then I throw the discussion open to the audience. Live REBT. I teach therapy that way to the public. And I do other workshops and live demonstrations as well, so I have helped innumerable professionals and members of the public with REBT.

I have also written over seventy-five books, more than eight hundred articles, and made two hundred cassettes. I have received thousands of letters from people who were helped by REBT all over the world. So my influence has been very wide and strong. Now that doesn't mean I have always succeeded. I am sure my detractors would say that I have even fallen short. But I like my accomplishments. However, I don't think that makes me a good person. I am okay whether or not I have the accomplishments, but it's great that I have them and I hope that I have helped change the field of psychotherapy considerably.

Q. You said that you wished you had done more research on REBT. Do you think that not having had that research makes it less influential today as compared to cognitive therapy as practiced by Beck?

A. Well, probably. But people, for example, use Meichenbaum's or Beck's cognitive behavior therapy, which are toned down versions of REBT without some of the best aspects of it. And one of the reasons they use them is because of the empirical studies that have been done on CBT. So, REBT has done less in terms of studies. But there are about 250 experiments using REBT showing that it works. So if therapists use REBT, and show clients how to find and give up their musts, they then do much of what is called cognitive behavior therapy today.

Q. Are people in your personal life, family, aware of the contribution you have made to the field of psychotherapy?

A. Well, my friends and relatives know my contributions because I am very well known. Many of them have read my books and listened to my cassettes. My own mother didn't (*smiles*). I used to send her my books but she did light reading, such as comics and magazines. She didn't read any books, including mine. So she knew vaguely what I did but not specifically. My brother was on our board of directors and helped us considerably. My father thought that REBT was quite okay.

Q. You mentioned that you started by doing a master's degree in psychology. Did you always intend to pursue psychology?

A. No, I got in by accident. I was training myself to be a writer. I originally got my BBA so that I could make good money and write anything I wanted. But then the Great Depression came along. And then accounting, which I majored in and was good at, was not my thing—I found it a bore. So I stopped that. I kept writing for years and had all kinds of jobs just to earn a living. But my writing wasn't selling, maybe it was too good, maybe it wasn't, but it wasn't selling. I wrote plays, novels, poems, you name it. I completed twenty full manuscripts by the age of twenty-eight. But then I decided that a good field was sex, love, and marriage, but nonfiction, not fiction. So I became an authority on love and sex. I read hundreds of books and articles on the topic and began writing articles. Then my friends and relatives heard about that and came to me for advice (*laughs*). And I found out to my surprise that in just a few informal sessions, I could help them with their sex, love, and marriage problems, show them what they were doing wrong, and tell them what to do instead. And I enjoyed that, so then at the age of twenty-eight, I went back to school and got my PhD in clinical psychology from Teacher's College, Columbia University.

Q. What projects are you involved in currently?

A. Well, I am currently revising some of my very popular books. *A Guide to Rational Living,* which sold over a million and a quarter copies when it first came out in 1961, is now being revised for the third edition. I am also revising another book that first came out in 1977, titled *Anger: How to Live with It and without It.* I am also revising a book for practitioners of therapy, called *The Practice of Rational Emotive Behavior Therapy,* which is being published soon. Finally, I am writing another book, titled *Rational Emotive Behavior Therapy Applied to Stress Counseling,* which is in press. Besides these projects, I am still continuing to write other articles and books. And I give many talks and workshops around the world

Q. For our professional readers, how would one go about obtaining training in REBT?

A. We have several training programs here, throughout the country, and all over the world. At the highest level, we offer one-year internships and two-year fellowships where the trainees attend workshops, receive supervision, and treat clients at our busy clinic. We only take about ten trainees a year. Then we have our briefer training programs where we start with three-day workshops and show professionals how to do REBT and then follow it up with advanced practicums where they bring in clinical tapes and receive supervision. So there are lots of training opportunities. People can also receive training and continuing education credits through the mail by listening to our cassettes and then sending us their clinical tapes.

Q. For consumers, when should they consider treatment with REBT? And how would they go about obtaining treatment with a therapist trained in REBT?

A. Consumers can write or call the Albert Ellis Institute in New York to find REBT therapists in their area. We have referral lists of therapists trained in REBT. I also do phone sessions with people who live outside of New York. People who live in the New York area can call and directly make an appointment with one of our Institute therapists or request a free catalog to see what programs we offer.

Q. How do you think you have personally benefited from REBT? You touched on that a little bit earlier. Do you apply it to yourself?

A. I benefited by devising some of the therapy and practices of REBT from reading and applying philosophy from the age of fifteen onward. By age nineteen, I got myself over some of my worst fears, such as a fear of public speaking and of encountering new women. I used what would later become the essence of REBT to overcome my anxiety, fearfulness, and hesitation and did very well. Now I am one of the best public speakers in the field and have no social or public speaking anxiety.

As can be seen from the material in this chapter, REBT started with my empirically based observations that many other therapies leave much to be desired and that helping people to help themselves has its main roots in philosophy and psychology. I think that I was innately philosophical *and* empirical from the start. These two integrated heads nicely serve REBT continually—as I hope the rest of this book will show.

NOTE

1. Reprinted from the *Realist* 16 no. 1 (March 1960): 9–14 and 17 (May 1960): 7–12. Revised 1983. Copyright © by the Albert Ellis Institute.

2

Core Philosophies
That People Use to
Disturb Themselves and That
They Can Radically Change

I have already described, in the first chapter and many of my other writings, the core philosophies that practically all people tend to often use to upset themselves and thereby create anxiety, self-deprecation, the damning of others, and their intolerance of life conditions. Let me now give the details of how I discovered them and saw what people can do, using REBT, to therapeutically change their thinking, emotions, and actions.

First, I observed my own self-defeating thoughts, feelings, and behaviors. I was never, as I remember, greatly self-downing, but I saw my errors and stupidities—my warts and flaws—fairly clearly and criticized them but not me, my whole person, for having them. Maybe I was raised, as a Reformed Jew, with little self-damnation. Maybe my mother was fairly forgiving. Maybe I imbibed self-acceptance from my vast reading of liberal novels, plays, and nonfiction. Anyway, when I did excoriate myself for my failings, I soon saw that it hardly helped me improve and often failed more when I saw myself as a *failure*. Self-castigation just didn't work, so I largely abandoned it. Being a natural pragmatist helped.

Particularly when I became a therapist at the age of forty-three, I fully saw that self-downing for one's errors and stupidities stopped practically all improvement and led to immense anxiety (in case one did fail) and depression (after one failed). No win!

I finally realized that all humans, me included, are highly fallible. Without fail. As I told in my book, *Rational Emotive Behavior Therapy: It Works for Me—It Can Work for You*, I dramatically forgave my sister, Janet, for her nastiness when I was fifteen. I later studied the followers of Lao-Tsu and Buddha, who were remarkably nonhostile. And I solidly learned about unconditional self-acceptance and unconditional other-acceptance (UOA) from Paul Tillich's *Courage to Be*, when I was already practicing therapy in 1953. That really worked—for my clients and for me.

I also realized—as Carl Rogers never seemed to do—that USA and UOA could not just be modeled by a therapist because clients turned them into *conditional* self-acceptance and conditional other-acceptance: "*Because* my therapist likes me and accepts me, I am therefore a good, worthy person." So I actively taught USA and UOA to my clients and helped them strongly teach them to themselves. That worked better!

I also *showed* my clients the virtues of USA and UOA and how *important* it was for them to adopt these philosophies. I *emotively* taught them to follow these core philosophies, and I *actively* encouraged them to *behave* in new ways.

I still find the achievement of UOA and USA very tricky. People sneak in *conditional* self-acceptance and other--acceptance even when they try to remove them. Thus, one of my clients recognized her putting *herself* and not just her *behavior* down when she was not *perfectly* competent. But she found herself praising her *self* and not just her *behavior* when she "perfectly" got temporarily rid of her perfectionism. She then considered herself "truly worthwhile." So she had to *im*perfectly succeed at unconditionally accepting herself before she got herself over this hill.

I, too, had to be alert to my *self*-lauding, instead of my activity-lauding, when I succeeded in fighting my self-damnation. That was really hard!

Can you really feel pride in your zapping your self-beration and still not praise your *self* for doing so? Yes, for a while. But you may frequently fall victim to *self*-praise—because it feels so good. Beware!

Recognizing your damning of *conditions* when they are vile but still not damning *the world* is also slippery. If parts of the world are *very* bad—such as sexually abusing children—isn't life itself "very rotten"?

No. *Parts* of it are "very rotten." But don't overgeneralize. *All* of life is not bad; its rotten parts may not last forever. Change is possible. Sometimes! If you give yourself unconditional life-acceptance (ULA).

Along with USA, UOA, and ULA, REBT holds that just about nothing is awful, terrible, or horrible—unless you think it is. Then, alas, you often *make* it so.

Of course, some things in life are bad, very bad, and even very, very bad. Floods, volcano eruptions, and hurricanes, for instance. Not to mention wars, torture, holocausts, and terrorism. But *awful* really means *totally* bad, as bad as it could be. But it could always be *worse*. Moreover, *terrible* means, "It's *so* bad that it *absolutely should not and must not exist*." But it *does*, factually, exist. And calling something *horrible* will tend to *make* less than totally bad things *seem* to be *worse* than they are. Exaggeration hardly helps *correct* bad events. Often *hinders* doing anything to better them.

Awful also implies that you positively *can't stand, can't bear* what is happening. But you rarely die of it—even war. And, if you think you *can* bear war, a holocaust, or grave illness, you can often find *some* happiness in spite of it, as many Holocaust victims managed to discover.

Other proofs of anti-awfulizing include relaxation and meditation techniques, of which there are quite a few. If you focus very strongly on watching your thinking, on saying, "Om, om, om," on imagined pleasures, or many other powerful distractions, you can minimize your awfulizing, at least for a time. Even physical pain can be shunted aside by these methods, while if you horribilize about it, it almost always intensifies.

Of course, you can kill yourself and thus avoid *awful* sufferings, and occasionally that may seem the lesser evil. But that is usually a little too final—and irreversible! *Awful* misery may come to an end while you are still alive and kicking. If you let it.

The main thing is that you usually have a *choice*. You may not stop very bad things from happening. But you can *choose* to refuse to awfulize about them. Look for the good things about them—for example, the death of a loved one releases him or her from pain. Or focus on anything else but "how *awful, terrible, and horrible* this affliction is!" Almost always that will increase its "horror."

Does the philosophy of REBT make *too little* of very bad events by minimizing awfulizing about them, and does it possibly reduce the human incentive to strongly push to improve them?

No, because it still holds that some—though only a few—things are *very* bad and merit concerted action to change them. Wars, for example, and holocausts. Why should we excuse and tolerate very bad events? But awfulizing tends to numb us, to make all action feel hopeless. Seeing things as very bad but not awful is more likely to help us work for improvement. Awfulizing rarely works. If anything, it may impede and dull our let's-take-action tendencies.

Awfulizing may also make things seem *so* bad that it is impossible to change them. This is perhaps what happened in Warsaw, when few of the restricted and downtrodden Jews did anything to make things better until very late in the game.

Conditional other-acceptance (COA) instead of UOA often first includes awfulizing about what others have done to "make" you discontented. It makes them the *origin* of your trouble—when, of course, they may have had little to do with "causing" it. "I would not have fallen had they not pushed me!" "I failed because the teacher gave me an unfair test!"

Second, you make your awfulizing damn *people*, not merely their *actions*: "Because they deliberately pushed me, which they *absolutely should not* have done, they are nasty, *no good people!*" Actually, they may have tried to help when they pushed you, and even if they were carelessly wrong, this was only *one* of their actions. When we awfulize, we cavalierly *overgeneralize* both their "wrongness" and their total selves for being wrong. Study Alfred Korzybski and his general semantics and see for yourself.

Of course, you have several nonawfulizing choices when adversity strikes you: (1) Live with it and do your best to remove it; (2) realize it is often inevitable; (3) see that it has some good aspects; (4) don't dwell on it and exaggerate its "horror"; (5) distinctly dislike it but still fully accept that it *should* exist (because it does) and often is an unfortunate but *partial* aspect of your life.

Anti-awfulizing, then, has many possibilities. Look out for them. See which one best suits you. Help other people interrupt their (common) awfulizing to help you see your own and preventively and alertly deal with it.

At the bottom of awfulizing often lies some unconscious perfectionism. For if bad things happen to you, it is frequently true that they *preferably* should not have happened to a "good person" like you, therefore are "quite unfair," preferably *should* change for the better, are "horrible," particularly if they last, and so on. But these are all highly unrealistic, hence perfectionistic, views. Because you intensely *dislike* them, they *must* not plague your life. Never! Your perfectionism is not only illogical—"Because I hate adversity, it must not exist!"— but it is also thoroughly antifactual. The real world is replete with happenings you definitely dislike and even frequently bring on. How could they *not* often occur?

Fortunately, misfortunes, difficulties, hassles, adversities, ailments, and unniceties occur—sometimes often—to all humans, including kings and queens, the well-to-do and rich, the talented and lucky, those with great and little support, people in good and poor circumstances. Not equally bad things, of course, but steady restriction of what they want and infliction of what they don't want. The human condition!

Very fortunately, however, as Epictetus showed two thousand years ago—it is not *only* the undesirable and uninvited things that happen to you that disturb you—it is *also* your view of them. Aristotle, too, wisely indicated that you could take unfortunate events lightly, moderately, or catastrophically. To a considerable degree, it's your *choice*. REBT, like several other constructivist therapies, gives you this choice and urges you to *wisely* select the best—meaning the most effective—for you, for other humans (and animals), and for the world. That is what wisdom seems to offer. But you have to keep working at using it. *See* your core philosophies and push your ass (PYA) to keep *using* them.

As you can see from the material in this chapter, REBT is philosophic in several important ways. Its general philosophy is that whatever unfortunate events and happenings exist in your (and, of course, others') life right now, they definitely *do* exist. They rarely can be *immediately* improved, and you had better accept—*gracefully*—what you cannot quickly change. To repeat, your accepting grim events means (1) fully acknowledging that they *should* exist when they do; (2) also acknowledging that people sometimes needlessly *make* them unfortunate; (3) and sadly determining that bad events will often exist, for you and others, but realizing that they *will* and there's no way of completely eliminating them. Too damned bad! But not *awful* or *horrible*. A real pain in the ass and a challenge to your potential strength *if* you sanely bear them while persisting in devising ways out.

3

Attempts To Take a Middle Road between Empirical Science and Spiritual and Religious Philosophies

For centuries, and especially in the last few decades, believers in spiritual and religious pathways have refused to accept "pure" empiricism although they have found no good arguments to refute it. Why this persistent espousal of nonempirical views and the efforts—sometimes frantic—to add spiritual-religious views of God and the world to them?

Religious views posit some kind of God or supernatural being. Spiritual but nonreligious philosophies omit God and the supernatural but hold that there is some mystical or semimystical essence to life that can never be explained with pure empirical or reality-oriented evidence. Many theories of "pure" spirituality and of spiritual mixed with empirical views have been invented. I stubbornly buy none of them. However, let me bend over backwards to show that these nonempirical (or semi-empirical) ways of looking at religion can also include some elements of "fact" or "reality" and can therefore be partially subscribed to by many skeptics.

WHY DO MANY PEOPLE IGNORE EMPIRICISM AND HOLD ON TO RELIGIOUS, SPIRITUAL, AND SOME SUPERNATURAL BELIEFS?

Even fairly skeptical people keep some elements of mysticism and anti-empiricism for several reasons, including these:

1. Devout religion and spirituality probably have biological, innate, and socially learned aspects. Probability and chance do not seem to be *enough* for many people, so they *invent* (highly improbable) certainty and feel comfortable with it. Only the gods can be *absolutely sure* of things. So we *assume* that certainty exists and we feel "safe" with this dubious assumption. Despite the fact that reality continually denies it and that we cannot have it in the ups and downs of factual living (which has innumerable vicissitudes), we feel secure—well, almost—in creating our own version of certainty. That "solves" our problem—temporarily. In fact, if we are dogmatically certain about certainty, we may indefinitely solve our problem of never *really* having it. Certainty seems to be axiomatic—though like all axioms, it is self-created and unprovable.

2. As Immanuel Kant showed, human knowledge increases over the years but will probably always be limited and restricted. Why are humans *really* here? What is their essential purpose? Will tomorrow's goals and ideals be written in stone? Even stone changes. We are allergic to fully facing these and other (perhaps millions) of unanswered questions. Some are unanswerable because we *change* our

future directions. Some questions—like "Can we be *certain* about our future?"—have a resounding no for an answer, for *certainty* means "for *all* time under *all* possible conditions." How can we be *absolutely sure* that our world, and *any* world, will survive? We can only say that it *probably* will or won't. Certainty may well be *intrinsically* uncertain.

3. We can always find many other people to join us in dogmas and certainties that cannot be empirically disproven. So religion and spirituality give us a sense of *belonging*. We are rarely *alone* in latching on to them. And since they really cannot be disproven, we can manage *never* to be alone. Attachment and sociality, as John Bowlby and others have shown, are partly acquired but also have a strong inborn factor (which helps preserve the human race). Again, they are "naturally" ingrained *and* acquired.

4. Nonspiritual skepticism includes the "spiritual" feelings of purposiveness, love, and joy—which, of course, many atheists have. In fact, spiritual feelings usually also include purposiveness, love, and joy. But again, though we can see that these feelings (usually) add much to our lives, how can we be *sure* they also have no disadvantages? *Can* we? Are the best of feelings—such as joy and love—completely worth it? Even if we can justifiably say, "Yes, they definitely are *today*," can we guarantee that they *will be* and *have to be* tomorrow?

Again, what is intrinsically "good" and, therefore, *forever* good? Values and ideas *often* change. If we agree on what is good, valuable, and worthwhile *now*, what assures our agreeing—the majority voting for it—in the future? Nothing!

5. Some serious ego problems arise to make us uncertain whether certainty or uncertainty can be accurately judged. If we face the "truth" and hold that absolute certainty would be very nice to have—because it would put all our major doubts to rest—then we feel deprived and weak (powerless to achieve it). Desirable things like certainty *should* exist, we conclude, so we never quite give up the search for such guarantees, and we go *un*certainly on looking, looking, looking. Since we never quite find certainty, we go wobblingly along. Even when we make it (temporarily) exist, by *defining* it a certain way (e.g., God certainly exists and his absolute rules for our living *have* to be true), our "certainty" is not empirically confirmable. Hence, we have no factual proof that certainty exists, and we still remain often in doubt—that is, uncertain that our definitions are absolutely confirmable. We still, consciously and unconsciously, look for observable—and therefore "real"—facts to make us sure of them. Ironically, only when we see, hear, sense, and *observe* God or his subjects and rules are we *sure* that our spiritual and religious inventions are "absolutely true." So, as much as we throw out all empirical "proofs" of spiritual beings, we finally tend to bring them back again.

We say that we "experience" God or "feel" his presence. But this seems to be a roundabout way of seeing that we somehow *see* that he exists. Our "seeing" him is really a delusion and is unconfirmable except by our strong *belief* that he *does* exist in the "real" (meaning observable) world. But our seeing, sensing, or experiencing God only (temporarily) *suffices* for the "real" deity, who is still unobservable.

On the other hand, if we honestly face uncertainty and godlessness, we once again face our inherent weakness in *not* having certainty; we often think that we *need* something supernatural to bring back the "certainty" we have just given up!

As long as we feel weak and powerless without certainty—which we often do—we either fully face its loss and are "nothing" unless we regain certainty, or we put ourselves down for "weakly" not having it and feel insecure and incomplete. We could solve this ticklish problem by honestly giving up (nonexistent) certainty and fully *accepting* our weakness and limitations in surrendering it. But for us humans to thus *accept* our weakness without berating ourselves for *having* it seems a most difficult thing to do. Accepting—without *liking*—our basic weaknesses itself seems to be "weak" and unforgivable. Impasse!

All of which brings me back to my own accepting philosophy of spirituality and religion. I think I am quite atheistic and empirical. I do not say that nothing supernatural exists or can exist. Maybe it does—but who cares? I see, sense, and feel only highly imperfect and limited humans and their imperfect environment. I wish that we (and it) were less imperfect—but still I fully accept that we aren't. So, with our limitations, we do our best to explain ourselves and the world—with no help from supernatural "forces" or "entities." Many things we honestly face are "weak" or "bad" limitations, but we still can *accept* them without liking them.

If we really do this, we don't eliminate real dangers because weaknesses lead to problems. But we eliminate most *ego dangers,* especially blaming *ourselves,* or self-rating, for our *limitations.* Yes, we have weak feelings, but we no longer beat ourselves for having them. As the saying goes, we accept ourselves for what we *are* with the weaknesses we inevitably have.

So our limitations—*human* limitations—remain, but not our flagellating ourselves for having them. We are, and admit we are, *very* fallible—as humans, not being gods, *should be.* By admitting this, we make ourselves much stronger. Atheistically resolute. Free from the ticklish problems of certainty and uncertainty. But though still saddled with uncertainty, we accept it and stop whining about it.

I could give several other reasons for our (false) *need* for perfect safety and the *additional* problems it gives us. But, really, our having a degree of probability that we won't let lack of certainty augment our life difficulties is enough. Probability isn't so bad—if we do not *think* it is! It might well be quite boring to live in a world filled with absolute knowledge of what the future may—or may not—bring.

4

Does Faith Actually Help Believers in Religious and Spiritual Philosophies to Improve Their Mental Health?

Some writers have for many years claimed that people's holding definite religious, supernatural, mystical, and spiritual views may admittedly sabotage their physical well-being and mental health. But they have meant that "bad" or "false" or "fraudulent" philosophies lead to this kind of outcome.

In the last few decades, the relationship of people's turning to religion and/or spirituality has received vastly increased attention and study; the consensus of almost innumerable articles and books in the field seems to be that "wrong" religious and spiritual views can hinder, while "good" ones may enhance people's physical and mental health and increase their happiness. At least *some* believers, especially disturbed ones, appear to benefit—or *say* they benefit—from their religious faith.

Much can be said for and against this allegation, for proreligionists can "discover" that a "spiritual" view bolsters mental health, and antireligionists can prejudicially "find" that it sabotages it. Who is to support unbiased claims in either direction? Virtually no one.

As I first pointed out almost forty years ago, self-ratings of how much you have benefited from *any* of your values are easily prejudiced by the values themselves. Thus, if you are conservative about marriage, you will often claim to researchers that your own marriage is "good" or "happy," while if you hold liberal views on marriage and divorce, you may more honestly tell researchers that your own marriage is "poor" or "unhappy." Many studies have shown—as I indicated in my 1965 critique, "The Validity of Personality Questionnaires"—that respondents who want to favorably impress researchers lie on their tests, while other respondents give more truthful answers when they are not ashamed of their more honest responses.

Almost all the many studies of the mental health of religious and nonreligious respondents are not to be trusted and may well be misleading. Most of them "show" that religious subjects say that they received definite benefits from following religious or spiritual attitudes—such as increased confidence, competence, productivity, and emotional well-being. They *say* they enhanced their lives, and most of them really believe that they did. But did they actually do so—or did they consciously and unconsciously exaggerate these "findings?" Who can accurately say? My guess—like that of many scientific researchers— is that many of the conservative respondents exaggerated the virtues of their religious attitudes and blithely ignored the disadvantages of either religious or spiritualized views.

Let me, however, give the Devil his due. Let me assume that many—perhaps millions—of people who say that religio-spiritual philosophies have enhanced their lives have distinctly benefited as they have reported. For one thing, their *thinking* they have benefited will often make their feelings valid. Thus, as I have mentioned before, if you devoutly *think* that Jesus or the Devil is helpfully on your side, even if this is only your delusion, you may *help yourself* by giving in to this delusion. As Shakespeare noted, "There's nothing either good or bad but thinking makes it so." Some of the worst delusions actually work. Moreover, if you are *profoundly convinced* that anything, including religious faith, will give you more confidence to do things, your *conviction* may lead you to *act* in a more productive way. People who *believe* that they can get a better job frequently push themselves and get one.

Let me assume that something beyond empiricism does exist and that your belief in this supernatural "thing" is not empirically justified or "true," but it helps you "spiritually" and awards you better mental and physical health and happiness. Assume that your religious or spiritual convictions are somehow "true"—that God or Jesus or Allah really does exist and your acknowledging his existence distinctly helps you live a "fuller" life.

Now try to assume the opposite: that there is nothing supernatural and no "spirits" in the world but that your *believing* that there are and worshipping the (false) dictates of a (nonexistent) deity somehow enhances your life—gives you, for example, a goal or purpose to live for.

In both these (conflicting) cases, you may win Pascal's wager—for you benefit either (1) by the existing God or (2) by the nonexisting but firmly dreamed of God. So what have you got to lose? You might as well *accept* God's existence—or not accept it but still act *as if* he existed.

This is what I think the majority of people do. They can't be sure that anything supernatural exists, but they also can't prove that it doesn't—so they choose to allege that because it *may* exist, it really does. They *choose* to be deists or theists. More skeptical people, however, choose to believe that supernatural beings most probably don't exist—since if they did, there would be *some* empirical evidence proving that they do—but they still retain some safety by acknowledging that they *may* possibly exist so they can accept their existence and still think it is possibly an illusion. Still more skeptical people think (as I do) that supernatural "things" most probably *don't* exist, so let's assume that they don't. Finally, dogmatic atheists believe that spiritual "things" absolutely don't exist and even *can't* exist. Apparently, people are able to *choose* their degrees of skepticism about spirits and gods.

Why do I choose to be a probabilistic atheist, who is *almost* certain that supernatural entities don't exist but nonetheless *may*? For several reasons:

1. Probabilistic atheism *most probably* is, as far as I (or any reasonable person) can *see*, factual or "true."
2. It is a non-safety-seeking, *honest* position to take. It represents *my* personal views.
3. It unbigotedly recognizes that gods, devils, and angels *could* possibly exist because even laws of probability are not *sacred*. Anything *could* happen even against the "laws" of probability.
4. Dogmatic, absolute atheism *is* unprovable and is a bigotry in itself, so I certainly don't want to subscribe to that.

5. Probabilistic atheism allows me—and others—to stop arguing about unprovable and undisprovable gods and get on with more important *life* problems. It saves needless discussion and bickering.
6. It accords with the *known* facts, keeps looking for the unknown ones, but doesn't obsess about them.
7. It enables me (and others) to *want* but not *need* perfectionism and certainty.
8. It surrenders the emotionally disturbed, sadistic, and very improbable idea that if there were gods, they would never forgive those of us who refuse to believe in them and roast us in hell forever. It paradoxically avoids making gods into human devils!
9. It gives me (and others) the freedom, the real freedom, to choose our own hypotheses, thoughts, feelings, and behaviors and to widen our possibilities of living.

I think that these are good reasons for keeping my probabilistically based atheism instead of some more caviling position. People denigrate me for holding it, but I can take their opposition without cringing.

Back to my question: Does faith actually help religious and spiritual people to improve their mental health? Yes, I'd better admit: With *some* gullible people it *sometimes* does. They think that they would be too uncomfortable taking the atheistic position that there is so little possibility of supernaturalism existing that they might as well *assume* that it does not—and they tell themselves, "I'll be safe and assume that supernatural entities *may* exist, that they may be helpful to me if they do, and that therefore I'd better believe in this and ask for their help." They then take a compromising, weak way out of this question, while people like me more honestly choose the atheistic way. If these middle-of-the-road compromisers are correct and there *is* a vengeful God who will punish nonbelievers, I'll risk taking that (improbable) consequence!

5

Using Rational Emotive Behavior Therapy with People Who Believe in Religion

U p until the year 2000, when I was eighty-seven years old, I was somewhat famous for my view that effective psychotherapy, such as REBT, was incompatible with firm religious conviction. As I have indicated in the previous chapter, I have been a staunch probabilistic atheist since I was twelve years of age. This means that I firmly believe that no gods or supernatural events, in all probability, do exist. But I am definitely open to the possibility that they *may exist* and importantly affect us humans. There seems to be no certain—or empirically confirmable—way for us to "prove" their nonexistence. Therefore, it seems folly to absolutistically hold that they *must* or *must not* be "real" or "true."

Belief in supernatural entities, which is one of the main attitudes of those who call themselves "religious" (or, sometimes, "spiritual" or "transcendental"), obviously is a "fact." One study after another has shown that the majority of people all over the world believe in some kind of religion and frequently practice the rules and rituals that go with it.

At first, in the 1960s, I tended to hold that virtually all

kinds of religious beliefs were mentally and emotionally harmful, because they contained some elements of one-sidedness, prejudice, dogma, bigotry, unreality, anti-empiricism, overgeneralization, needless restriction, and other interferences with human "rights" and happiness. Particularly in regard to the humanistic view of what goals and purposes they preferably should hold to foster their well-being, freedom, and creativity, I said that religious-minded people were self-sabotaging and socially destructive and would be better off if they freed themselves of all vestiges of faith unfounded on fact.

I then realized that I was being too harsh and prejudiced myself. As Allen Bergin pointed out in his article "Psychotherapy and Religious Values," and as W. Bradford Johnson, Stevan Nielsen, and many other psychologists and writers have been showing in reputable journals, there are many different kinds of religious views and values—a large number of which distinctly differ from each other. "Religion" is multifaceted and ranges from liberal and moderate attitudes to strict, fundamentalistic, and fanatical philosophies and practices. My placing virtually all religious and supernatural attitudes under one omnibus heading made me resort to overgeneralizing, which Alfred Korzybski soundly criticized and saw as a main source of human evil. I was therefore contradicting Korzybski, whom I have supposedly agreed with and incorporated into REBT since the 1950s. How careless of me!

Accordingly, I revised my first major article, "The Case against Religion," in 1983 and retitled it "The Case against Religiosity." In this revised version—as well as in my 1973 book, *Humanistic Psychotherapy: The Rational Emotive Approach*—I loosened up considerably in my opposition to religion. I defined "religiosity" as (1) "a devout or orthodox belief in some kind of supernatural religion" or (2) the pious adherence to a devout belief in some kind of secular religion (such as libertarianism, Marxism, or Freudianism).

In other words, I included in the word *religiosity* an absolutistic secular conviction that some political, social, or philosophic view is sacrosanct, provides ultimate answers to virtually all important questions, and is to be piously subscribed to and followed by everyone who wishes to lead a "good" life.

This was quite different from my former view, since it placed the emphasis for *both* supernatural and secular religion on rigidity and absolutism rather than on "religion" itself. I said in my revised paper that REBT held "religious" and "secular" values as "healthy" as long as they included self-interest, self-direction, social interest, tolerance, acceptance of ambiguity, acceptance of reality, commitment, risk-taking, and self-acceptance. These values came close to my recommended goals, which I keep stating in this book, for human mental health—including (1) unconditional self-acceptance, (2) unconditional other-acceptance, and (3) unconditional life-acceptance.

Even that did not thoroughly get religion quite off the hook, so in 1997 I gave still more thought to this problem of religion and mental health and began to give more credence to several practitioners of REBT who integrated it with their clients' religious outlook. They held that several REBT values and philosophies were remarkably similar to some

Judeo-Christian attitudes and therefore enhanced the mental health of the religious believers who subscribe to them. At the same time, some REBT practitioners included in their practice the *teaching* of several specific religious and spiritual philosophies *along with* REBT methods and held that the combination of the two techniques aided personality change and emotional health.

Thus, articles and books advocating the use of REBT together with some form of pastoral counseling include publications by Raymond DiGiuseppe, Mitchell Robin, and Windy Dryden; Paul Hauck; W. Bradford Johnson; C. Lawrence and Charles Huber; Lily Kemmler; Stevan Nielsen; Hank Robb; and Howard Young. All these REBTers include religious elements, though each one does it somewhat differently. They also report that using REBT religiously, especially when it is combined with Judeo-Christian attitudes, often works very well.

Why is putting REBT within a religious context at times so effective, although my first opinion predicted harm rather than good in doing so? Giving this matter more serious consideration helped me come up with some likely hypotheses.

Religious views include faith in supernaturalism—that is, faith unfounded on fact—but also include many practical maxims and practices that can definitely be tested and found effective. The Judeo-Christian code, for example, says, "Love thy neighbor as thyself" and "Condemn the sin but not the sinner." A number of nonreligious sayings—such as many marriage and family propositions—essentially agree. Why? Because the opposite rule, "Damn the sin *and* the sinner!" has been tried in various cultures and has led to relatively poor results. People were, perhaps, less sinful in these cultures, but they were often more panicked and depressed. Therefore, these moral dictates didn't work too well, and more effective philosophies were substituted for them.

Another hypothesis: the religions and the prevailing cultures that commonly feature philosophies of damning people who "sin" and of encouraging them to damn themselves for their religious and other infractions often encouraged rage and self-downing that eventually led to sinners upsetting themselves. Thus, they may have been (consciously or unconsciously) angry at the restrictive sinful rules, at the religionists who impose them, or at themselves for not following stern restrictions. Or they may have followed the rules against "sinning" but had low frustration tolerance about missing out on the pleasures they would have had if these depriving rules didn't exist.

Several possibilities, mostly leading to considerable frustration, anger, anxiety, and depression, are likely. When people in a Judeo-Christian, Muslim, or other pleasure-limiting culture feel holier than thou because they choose to avoid "sinning," and thereby are "rewarded" for doing so, they reap distinct emotional "gains" of an ego-satisfying nature. But their "gains" simultaneously include taking on needless frustration and pains. Don't they?

If restricting religious and "moral" rules are viewed as being "too strict," they will often be theoretically "accepted" but actually carried out poorly—or not carried out at all. If so, the strict rules of the people in some cultures will tend to be neglected or modified, and the religious fanaticism of the people of those cultures may wane. Or it may even be replaced by extreme hedonism—as supposedly happened in Sodom and Gomorrah. Or some religious cultists may find life "useless" or "worthless" and may resort—as in Guyana, western Switzerland, and California—to mass suicide.

My main point still stands: Fanatical religionists may have a tendency—because of people's not-to-be-denied hedonistic nature—to eventually be lax and let their strict rules die out. Their self-imposed super-restrictions may defeat themselves and be replaced by less fanatical laws and rituals. Comes the revolution—and ultimately comes the counterrevolution!

I repeat: For reasons such as those discussed in the preceding paragraphs, devotees of fanatically restrictive religions that last for a while may eventually adopt less fanatical views and become run-of-the-mill religionists. If so, the laws and rules that implement their fanaticism may give way to "more reasonable" and "reformed" dictates—as has happened with several highly austere rules that have, over the centuries, become much less austere. Of course, the opposite may happen, too: As people in a certain culture become less fanatical about their religious rules, they may get bad results. Those who ban eating pork, for instance, may first ignore that ban, then may start getting diseased, and may then enforce stricter bans.

I still would guess, however, that fanatical religious (and nonreligious) restrictions will often prove to be too onerous for many people's low frustration tolerance and pleasure-seeking and will therefore often be relaxed. This will sometimes lead to less difficult and more "sensible" rituals. In the long run, what works, works—and may tend to become more common. Thus, several researchers have found that religious people who view God as a warm, caring, and lovable friend rather than as a punishing dictator and tyrant and who see religion as supportive, are significantly more likely to stay free from substance abuse than those who take a more negative view of God. When I reviewed the studies on religion in 1997 and saw that religious and academic researchers—like Lee Kirkpatrick, Richard Gorsuch, and others—presented this evidence, I took another look at religion and mental health and began to see, first, that liberal and moderate religious believers could sometimes be happier and healthier than fanatical ones, and, second, that some people who strongly and devoutly hold religious views could also benefit from holding them.

This, of course, seems to be obvious in the case of some religionists who powerfully believe that irreligious forces—such as the Devil—will frequently drive people to drink, gamble, and even murder. Believing this, these devout upholders of negative religious views rigorously stay away from various kinds of "sin." Some of them, for example, who believe that sex is "evil" and will lead them to hell, remain abstinent all their lives! But some people who fanatically believe that a kind, loving God will protect them from "evil" masturbation and fornication also manage to remain abstinent. Here we have two sets of people who rigorously refuse to give into their "normal" urges to engage in sexual "sin" for radically different religion-based reasons!

The powerful influence of religious beliefs, both pro and

con, has been pointed out for many years, especially by scientists who take a negative view of faith that has no empirical backing. Just a few of the noted skeptics who have held that fanatical religion is likely to harm people include Heywood Broun, Charles Darwin, Edward Gibbon, Thomas Huxley, Robert Ingersol, Thomas Jefferson, Paul Kurtz, Madeleine Murray, Friedrich Nietzsche, Bertrand Russell, Carl Sagan, Albert Schweitzer, Edward Wilson, and many more.

An impressive crew—some of whom persuaded me to adopt firm probabilistic atheism just before I reached adolescence. I think I was guided not by their reputations but by their sensible empirical arguments. Nonetheless, after firmly showing the harm of fanatical religiosity for many years, I finally accepted in 1997 the proposition that even devout religious faith *could* benefit a good many believers. It often didn't; it frequently had its destructive aspects. But it wasn't always "bad," and it sometimes included distinct advantages.

Naturally, especially as a therapist, lecturer, workshop presenter, and writer, I asked myself, "*Why* do some religious philosophies result in advantages and benefits—and some don't?" Following REBT, I answered, "Because they take the same stance as many secular philosophies that also aid mental and emotional health." As I have noted in this book, what we call people's outlook, attitude, value system, point of view, or cognitive assessment is, in large part, the answer. REBT naturally holds that people's *feelings and actions* also, combined with their thinking, makes them mentally healthy or unhealthy. The environment in which they were raised and their genetic inheritance also significantly contribute to their outlook. *Many* factors, which strongly *interact* with one another, "cause" or "create" cognitive, emotional, and behavioral processes.

However, one aspect of their thinking, feeling, and doing that people can often clearly observe and work at changing is their thinking. This can be translated into language—for example, "I see that my thoughts are getting me or not getting me what I want." Inner language can sometimes be quickly and effectively changed. Thus, "My thought that God will punish me if I drink, take drugs, or have sex" can be changed to, "The God in which I choose to believe is a warm, caring, and forgiving God who will accept me as a sinner and encourage and help me to change."

Once you change your religious thinking in this new direction, you will (1) more easily think, "My God and I can accept me even with my sins," (2) *feel* less blame and guilt, and (3) continue to *practice* new behaviors. So changing your religious (nonaccepting) destructive thinking won't automatically *make* you less disturbed. But it may appreciatively help! That is why the *way* you religiously think is quite important. Reviewing the connection between your attitude and your mental health and correcting attitudes that encourage disturbance is effective in *both* religion and psychotherapy.

Having hinted at the overlapping of religious philosophies and the REBT views that frequently aid mental health, let me be specific and list some of their main agreements. I shall mainly use the Judeo-Christian views that are similar to the tenets of REBT, but illustrations of Muslim, Buddhist, Taoist agreements can easily be found. Moderate and devout believers in many religions often tend to endorse some of the seminal REBT attitudes. Here are some examples:

- *REBT Philosophy of Unconditional Self-Acceptance*: I can rate my thoughts, feelings, and behaviors as "good" or "effective" when I and other people see that they lead to beneficial or unbeneficial results. But I cannot accurately give a global or general rating to my *self* or *personhood* because I do thousands of tasks and projects during my lifetime, many "good" and many "bad." I can always give myself unconditional self-acceptance and see myself as a "worthy" individual who deserves a happy and productive life. I can unconditionally accept myself just because I choose to do so—because I am alive and human. I will try to act well and win people's cooperation and approval, but I don't *have to* do so to prove my worth as a person. When I achieve my goals and purposes, I shall think that *that* is good but not that *I* am a good *person*. I shall try to desist from this kind of inaccurately *over*generalizing.
- *Religious Philosophy of Unconditional Self-Acceptance*: I am a fallible, imperfect child of God, who will keep making some serious mistakes. My God is merciful and will always accept me as a sinner while urging me to be less sinful. Because my God accepts me unconditionally in spite of my failings, I can and will fully accept myself as a good person in his eyes and in my own life.
- *REBT Philosophy of Self-Control and Personal Improvement*: I have a tendency to often avoid self-disciplined behaviors

that will help me and others today and tomorrow. I weakly demand that I absolutely must have immediate gratification and must avoid discomfort. But I can discipline myself, give up my short-range "necessities," and make myself seek present pleasures that will not harm me today or tomorrow. Although it is often hard, I can pursue my healthy short-range and long-range interests.

- *Religious Philosophy of Self-Control and Personal Improvement:* God gave me a considerable degree of free will and the ability to think for myself and to control my harmful immediate gratifications. With God's help, I can stop my self-harming activities. God helps those who help themselves.

- *REBT Philosophy of Unconditional Other-Acceptance:* Like me, all humans are quite fallible and will rarely become less fallible when I angrily criticize them. If I blame them for their misdeeds, they will often damn me back and refuse to change their ways. If anything, they may act worse. I had better realistically accept people with their errors and their wrongdoings and encourage them to correct their behavior. Hating harmful, angry people will frequently induce them to defensively deny the wrongness of their acts and will help them revengefully increase it. Therefore, I had better unconditionally accept them as fallible humans, deplore their sinning, and not damn them as hopeless sinners.

- *Religious Philosophy of Unconditional Other-Acceptance:* My God and my religion encourage me to love my neighbors and other wrongdoers, to pray for them, and to try to help them reform. Blessed am I if I am merciful and forgive the sinners but not their sins. Judge not, that ye be not judged.

- *REBT Philosophy of Unconditional Life-Acceptance and High Frustration Tolerance:* Life inevitably includes many misfortunes and distresses for practically everyone. Some conditions are moderately bad, some very bad, and a few exceptionally bad. When I experience unfortunate conditions, I shall do my best to improve them. But if I assess them as *awful, terrible,* or *horrible,* I imply that they are *totally* bad, as bad as they *could* possibly be, and that I *can't stand* them and manage to be happy *at all.* My exaggerated, overgeneralized evaluation of unfortunate happenings will tend to paralyze me and keep me from trying to correct them. It will often make bad things seem *hopeless and unchangeable.* It frequently will *stop* me from coping with them and finding some enjoyment in my life in spite of them. Therefore, I'd better accept misfortunes that I cannot change and find some enjoyable pursuits in spite of them. Bad events don't make *everything* bad— unless I *see* them that way.
- *Religious Philosophy of Unconditional Life Acceptance and High Frustration Tolerance:* God cares for me and will help me to weather and cope with real misfortunes. If I trust in God and uncomplainingly accept life's tribulations, I will deal much better with them. God's will be done. In time, God will help me resolve my worst problems, for I have learned to find resources in myself whatever my circumstances.
- *REBT Philosophy of Achieving Major Goals and Purposes and Winning the Approval of Significant Others:* I distinctly prefer to achieve my major goals and purposes and to win the approval of significant others, but I never have to

accomplish these desires to prove that I am a worthwhile person. I will always accept myself as worthy whether or not I am achieving and lovable. Success and approval of others are desirable but not necessary.

- *Religious Philosophy of Achieving Major Goals and Purposes and Winning the Approval of Significant Others:* I am a good person merely because God loves me. Therefore, I don't have to accomplish my major goals and purposes and don't have to be approved by significant others. God's love will help me succeed and be lovable. If I am worthy of his love, that by itself makes me worthwhile. What does it profit a man if he gains the whole world but ruins or loses himself?

- *REBT Philosophy of Personal Choice and Free Will:* Although my past social conditioning has some influence over how I think, feel, and act, and although my heredity also influences and restricts me in important ways, I still have a good measure of free will or personal choice and can exert considerable control over what I do and do not do. Although my past may still partially affect my life, it need not seriously affect me forever. I can distinctly improve my life today and tomorrow and control much of my destiny. I am not completely ruled by my past.

- *Religious Philosophy of Personal Choice and Free Will:* God has granted me a good measure of personal choice and free will and has given me the option of using it. I am influenced but not irrevocably bound by my history. If I follow God's will, the old order has gone and a new order has already begun for me.

- *REBT Philosophy of Accepting My Own Disturbances:* I live in a stressful world and am born and reared with a tendency to neurotically react to its stresses and misfortunes. I also can make myself anxious, depressed, and enraged about my disturbability and thereby bring about double-headed disturbance. But I have the ability to accept (while disliking) my neurotic proneness and to refuse to damn myself for this weakness. If I refuse to blame my *self* but only dislike my disturbability, I will have a much better chance to minimize it.
- *Religious Philosophy of Accepting My Own Disturbance:* God is merciful and undamning. He will accept me with my neurotic disturbances and help me to relieve them. With his love, I can accept myself even when I make myself disturbed, and I can stop myself from adding to my neurotic behavior.

If you carefully consider the above similarities between REBT and religious-oriented philosophies and rules of conduct, you can see how close they often are. Not that they are exactly alike! But I think that many followers of REBT and firmly held religious outlooks will feel comfortable and unconflicted in adopting both these formulations. Perhaps the REBTers will have more unconditional acceptance of themselves (USA), of other people (UOA), and of life's inevitable difficulties (ULA). But some religionists will not lag far behind in these respects.

You will find many examples of how people and their therapists can use combined REBT and religious attitudes in my book with Stevan Nielsen and W. Bradford Johnson, *Counseling and Psychotherapy with Religious Persons.*

6

The Dangers of Extreme, Absolutistic, and Fanatic Religious and Spiritual Philosophies

Although I have acknowledged, in the previous chapter, that if you take a compromising, middle-of-the-road attitude toward religion and spirituality, you may derive more physical and emotional benefits than disadvantages, I have not yet dealt with extreme attitudes that *un*compromising religionists frequently hold. You can guess that I believe that such extreme views often do *some* good but that this is usually outweighed by the distinct harm that they wreak and that REBT is designed to reduce.

Here again we have a ticklish question that cannot be completely resolved. When I call religio-spiritual views extreme or fanatic, that is fairly well understood. Thus, if people are against giving a woman an abortion because they think that fetuses have a right to life, they hold a "regular" right-to-life view. But if they hold that a pregnant—and perhaps raped—woman carrying a diseased child that will kill her unless she quickly has an abortion still should not be allowed to have one, we can reason that their view is fanatic and extreme.

Okay, but we still would have trouble in holding that extreme views always produce much harm and little good. *Why* is an abortion that saves the life of a pregnant woman always "good," and why is that same abortion that ends the life of a diseased fetus always "bad"? *Some* good and bad results may occur in both cases—and not *always* agreed upon by "moral" people.

Let me take a prejudiced stab at contending that my view of "good" and "bad" results is "right"—which I can hardly inconvertibly contend. Admitting my prejudices, however, I can then "legitimately" hold that certain fanatical religious and spiritual attitudes appear to do a great deal more moral and social harm than the same views that are not fanatically, but only nonfanatically, held. Here, for example, are some fairly typical extreme views that appear to me—and many other nonextreme people— to create more social harm than good. Maybe in heaven they lead to great good. But hardly on this earth!

1. Devout Jews, Catholics, Muslims, and other religionists often fanatically hold that they are God's *specially chosen* people and are therefore *better* than other people. Arrant egotism! Why should God choose them? What prejudice! How does God's view, if he is one-sided enough to have it, *make* religionists outstanding? Won't it encourage them to denigrate all nonchosen people and to fight with them to retain their *special* privileges? Isn't designating your own group as "special" and other groups as "inferior"

incredibly (and without any confirming evidence) misleadingly self-centered and undeservedly super-worthy?

2. If God "specialized" members of one religion for their past deeds—for example, their devout attachment and allegiance to him—why should their "superiority" *always* remain? Don't they have to *do* something to *maintain* his good graces? What?

3. "I am lovable and forgivable because God (and his son, Jesus) loves *everyone*." Why is God so indiscriminate? How does his loving me and others *make* us lovable people in *all* respects? What makes his indiscriminateness sacred and holy? Why must I accept God's opinion?

4. "The more significantly human we are, the more we reveal the meaning of divinity and make ourselves divine." How is our *humanity* equated with our divinity? Since we are exceptionally *fallible*, and God is not, isn't this contradictory?

5. Some religions, like Buddhism, are really atheistic. Yet Buddhists deify and worship the Buddha!

6. "Religious faith and prayers for you, even if you are unaware that others have it, can cure your physical and mental problems." How miraculous! Your own faith in healing may possibly help you. But *other people's* faith that you don't even know exists? You can prove that they have it, but how do you know that their faith alone really helped you?

7. If women of some orthodox religions—for example,

Muslims—reveal any parts of their bodies in public, that makes them thoroughly bad and punishable— even by death. Their God presumably spies on them continually and *makes* them into *bad people*, even if they are innocent of any other wrongs.

8. Some religious devotees, like extreme Zen Buddhists, have to reach Nirvana and give up *all* desire to achieve holiness. But obviously, if they achieved complete desirelessness, they wouldn't want to eat and survive.

9. Many fanatical religionists believe that there is no morality, no justice, no honesty without their believing in a divine power. But atheists obviously have *some* morality, justice, and honesty without such a belief. Did God grant it to them in spite of their nonbelief?

10. Passionate defenders of the right to life oppose killing a fetus even to save the life of the pregnant mother because the Catholic Church (for instance) makes this rule. But how can we know that God would *always* follow this rule, even if he originally recommended it? Maybe he sometimes relents and follows a more merciful rule.

11. The Bible can be taken literally, as *divine word* always to be followed—or as R. L. Fox and other Christians have suggested, as *human truth*. But human truth is not invariant and to some degree depends on exceptionally varied conditions and circumstances. Does it rigidly exist as truth no matter *what* conditions exist?

12. Certainty-based physical and emotional cure

knows "the best" religious treatment for *all* ailments. It is held to be "the only way," as posited in devout Christian Science. Even if it were "*among the best*," why couldn't it be used *along with* certain medical procedures?

13. An austere, stringent practice of Islamism is rigidly opposed to *bida*—any modernization that deviates from the fundamentalist teachings of the Koran. Moslem opposition to *bida*, like fundamentalist Christianity, is *certain* that any deviation or modernization is false and pernicious. Since deviation and modernization are accepted in virtually all other human affairs—like politics and economics—how can fundamentalists *be sure* that they can't work in religion?

14. Fundamentalist religion uses excommunication as well as regular restriction to enforce its rigid views. Thus, Catholic fundamentalists have excommunicated members of several groups—such as Planned Parenthood and Catholics for a Free Choice—in Nebraska and other regions. Excommunication is a drastic form of restriction on human's *choice* of what groups they want to ally with. Their preferences are entirely taken away from them—which appears to be more than a little fascistic.

15. Fundamentalism in religion encourages fraud and lying about important things, including historical events. Thus, modern archaeological and biblical research has revealed that the "evidence" for the existence of Abraham and Moses is spurious and that the

tumbling of the walls of Jericho never occurred. Religious "truths" can be very misleading!

16. Fundamentalist rigidity may obliterate people's most useful and freedom-loving propensity—to exert and sharpen their ability to think for themselves. Thus, Supreme Court Justice Antonin Scalia has said, "A person's religious faith is something that he or she must take whole from the church doctrine and obey." This is essentially what fascistic governments say: "A person's political and economic view is something that he or she must take whole from the state's doctrine and obey." Where art thou, freedom to think for oneself?

17. Fundamentalism in religion attributes to God and the supernatural many unusual but still very natural events that have nothing to do with deities—and that even could be seen as the Devil's intervention. Thus, when a girl was in a semicomatose state and could hardly influence anyone, thousands of people lined up to get close to her and her "saintliness" and benefit from the contact.

18. A poll conducted by *Newsweek* revealed that 66 percent of all adults believe in the Devil and more than one-third claim to have been tempted by him. Why was he silent about tempting the rest of us?

19. Dr. M. Y. Shapkle was sentenced to death in Pakistan for blasphemy against the prophet Mohammed. First of all, Mohammed has been dead for years. Second, even if he were alive, why would he take

criticism so seriously? What made him so supersensitive to mere words?

20. Cult members actually commit suicide en masse because their leaders tell them to do so. In 1997, for example, thirty-nine cult members killed themselves, demonstrating another example of organized madness. In western Switzerland, forty-eight members of the Solar Temple cult killed themselves "to escape hypocrisy expressed in this world."

21. Israeli police reported more than six incidents in which ultraorthodox Jews attacked women whose dress they considered immodest or provocative.

I could go on and on with similar or worse examples of religious and spiritual fanaticism. This hardly proves that most religionists are one-sided fanatics, are severely disturbed, and create considerable harm. The great majority of moderate, middle-of-the-road religionists are not rabid or destructive. Obviously, they are not arrant usurpers of other people's freedom. There is considerable evidence that they help rather than harm others.

But! The danger always remains that even the moderate and middle-of-the-road religionists may begin to think and act in extreme ways, such as some of those listed above. Who is to stop them? Only their own saner proclivities—if they have them!

I maintain, in this and my other books on REBT treatment, that just about *all* humans are easily self-disturbable and take other people and their ways *too* seriously. I also think that fanatical religious and spiritual people are *more* disturbable than nonreligious and semireligious people. They *more* often take their views to fanatical extremes because, I suspect, that is one of the basic (biological and socially conditioned) attitudes of religious fundamentalists. They are extreme in their dismissal of many harsh realities of the world—including God's failure to take special care of them. So they take a Pollyannaish view—that beneficial gods do definitely exist—and refuse to acknowledge that this possibility is highly unlikely. Then it is easy for them to see that the supernatural constructions that they invent also sadistically sanction the persecution of people who fail to rigidly follow God's noble rules. Coincidentally, these sacred rules are similar to the whims and prejudices of many actual rule makers—extremist and fanatic fundamentalists.

One more reminder. As noted throughout this book, people can honestly hold views and "laws" that are well intentioned but that lead to much human harm. With so many possible regulations to subscribe to and millions of people to favor one set of "good" rules and millions of dissenters to endorse "bad" rules, widespread differences will prevail. These appear to stem largely from their "human nature." Permit yourself these differences and don't regret them. Life goes on and presumably will continue in spite of them. But consider the rigidity and fanaticism with which you—and many others—are prone to foist your indubitably "beneficial" commands on those who don't choose to believe in and follow your "commands from heaven." Check your dogmatism, certainty-seeking, rigidity, and obsessive-compulsive *insistence* on "persuading" others to follow your rules and restrictions. Isn't that a basic issue in your choosing of "right" and "wrong" religious, political, social, and other behavior? It is not just *what* you choose to believe and not believe in—for it is unlikely that you will have no beliefs or completely neutral ones. Belief is one of the main and very important aspects of our "human nature." It also adds challenge and absorption. So keep your beliefs, views, attitudes, and philosophies much less rigidly than you—like other people—are prone to do. Let belief without fanaticism be your choice.

7

My Prejudices about Encouraging Religious Philosophies and Practices

As I have shown so far in this book, having profound religious faith benefits the mental health and happiness of many people but also may develop into one-sided dogma and fanaticism that is antihumanistic and harmful. Because people have many kinds of religiousness and follow its teachings in radically different ways, and because we humans cannot yet agree on what is absolutely "right" and "wrong"—meaning "beneficial" and "harmful" to most of us most of the time—we have difficulty in evaluating the "effectiveness" of religious beliefs.

This goes not only for theological religions (like Judaism, Christianity, and Islam) that posit supernatural gods but also for secular religions (like fascism and Nazism) that raise political, social, and economic philosophies to absolutistic extremes and deny any usefulness to opposing views. Both secular and God-involved religions have their fanaticism and their dangers; that is why in 1968 I wrote *Is Objectivism a Religion?* to show that Ayn Rand's philosophy is fanatically rigid, impractical, antihumanistic, and potentially harmful. I have recently revised this book under the title *Ayn Rand: Her Fanatical Religious and Fascistic Philosophy*.

I now see, however, that I hold my views about religion and spirituality strongly and passionately—perhaps *too* passionately. My "right" humanistic attitudes, which I have had since the beginning of my adolescence, are also very strong and solidly set—as those of many humanists, social revolutionists, and do-gooders probably are. Supposedly, we *seem* to base our views on empirically backed hypotheses—that if our favorite humanistic (and Bill of Rights) espousals were generally implemented, unusually "good" results would ensue. But we are *emotionally* as well as *scientifically* convinced of the "goodness" of our propositions, and we do not take too seriously the possibility that we may be wrong. Again, we passionately—perhaps too passionately—believe what we believe and conclude that our beliefs *surely* are valid.

I have for almost fifty years held that our thoughts, feelings, and behaviors are not disparate—as most people still seem to believe—but are intrinsically, interactionally, and integrally connected. When we *think*, we also feel and behave. When we *feel*, we also think and behave. When we *behave*, we also think and feel. When our bodies and brains function normally, thinking-feeling-behaving is our nature, created by our heredity *and* our environmental social learning.

If I am right about this, we'd better fully acknowledge that our beliefs are often partly "objective" or "dispassionate"—such as: "I'd better wait for a green light before I cross the street because it is dangerous if I don't." This belief is realistic and is based on empirical "facts." It also includes emotion because I *desire* to preserve my life. But largely it is based on "facts" regarding traffic, green lights, accidents, my physical vulnerability, and so forth.

Suppose, however, my *profound conviction* is, "All traffic is terribly dangerous, and none of the cars on the street is to be trusted at all. Oh, my God!" With this sort of strongly held, *emotional* conviction, I may never try to cross the street and may stop practically all my movement.

My main point remains. At present, REBT and most other psychotherapies follow humanistic procedures, for therapy consists of caring for and helping people. But, as I have attempted to show, most religions are also considerably caring and humanistic. That is why I am no longer strongly opposed to religion and why I now think that many aspects of faith unfounded on fact can be used with REBT and other cognitive therapies.

I hold this view, ironically, because of my strong faith in empiricism and my strong lack of faith in anything unfounded in fact. As an empiricist, I believe that no matter how strongly I (and others) "know" that supernatural entities most probably don't exist, I also "know" that they would "explain" unusual experiences and other "mysteries" if they did exist. But my solid empirical prejudices against supernaturalism, which have an emotional element ("faith founded in fact simply *has to be* superior to groundless faith"), make me "sure" about this hypothesis. This is almost opposite to the emotional element of true believers in the supernatural. ("I know every mystery *doesn't* have to have a magical explanation, but I am 'sure' that some of them do have one.")

My "emotional" attachment to naturalism cannot be upheld by pure empirical reasoning because, like most emotions, it is really based on strong conviction rather than provable fact. But its very strength makes me suspect that I am following my *desire* that nothing supernatural exists, and desires are emotional and do not totally follow from conclusions based on facts.

The question, then, is "Why do I so strongly (emotionally) *desire* that supernaturalism, transcendentalism, and gods and all their trappings be nonexistent?" Why don't I take the evidence that many people's *belief* in religion, but not unverifiable supernatural things *themselves*, is helpful?

My moderate belief that religious faith has some advantages and can be helpful to some people seems open-minded. But my prejudice against combining REBT and religious faith also has distinct emotional elements.

I have had this emotionalized belief ever since I first became a probabilistic atheist. I believe that there is *so* little chance of anything supernatural existing that I *assume* this is true. Because I strongly believe this, I *desire* to hold this assumption. So I'd better admit that in having this belief, I am also emotional about it.

Why do I emotionally believe that nothing supernatural exists and that I and others had better accept this "fact"? For several reasons, including these:

1. I—and others, if they agree with me—can definitely get on with our lives without wasting time debating whether supernatural forces exist and can help us. Let's assume that they are unavailable and get right on with our lives.

2. If we don't rely at all on God's help or some other supernatural force, we can devote our full attention to what *we* and any natural forces can do to help ourselves. The less we believe in supernatural forces, the more we will tend to believe that *we* can handle things without their intervention. This gives us more confidence and responsibility for looking for ways out of our dilemmas.

3. Many of us believe in God because we think he will punish us if he does exist and he discovers that we *don't* believe in him. This view sees God as a damner—which is a negative belief because that hardly helps our mental health. It may encourage us to damn ourselves and other people.

4. Belief in God's helpfulness may imply that we are not *able* to meet life's adversities and cope with them. Then we may not try to do as much coping as we really are able to do.

5. It is somewhat dishonest and weak to assume that if natural forces cannot help us, religious and magical forces can do the trick. It encourages our giving up instead of continuing to look for solid, empirically oriented ways of improving ourselves and the conditions we live under.

6. If there really are no absolutely certain ways of dealing with our lives and with world Adversities, we had better accept this grim fact, deplore it but not awfulize about it, and get on with this difficult life. Our realistic acceptance of not being able to change some Adversities is

not likely to occur while we still unrealistically believe that God and supernatural forces are somehow available to provide miracles. If we think that supernormal forces will give us a missing limb or make us grow younger, nonaccepting attitudes about our handicaps will block us from making the most of the advantages we still have.

7. Our stubborn, head-in-the-sand refusal to accept presently unchangeable difficulties adds to our low frustration tolerance (LFT) and cry-babyness. It is a weakness of our character and a defensiveness about stoically and uncomplainingly acknowledging our human limitations. Our LFT then makes us still weaker and less prone to change the many unniceties that we can change. It encourages procrastination and stick-in-the-mud behavior.

8. If believing in gods and supernatural spiritual entities really enhances our mental health, it does so because we have faith in the helpfulness of these nonobservable spirits. But we then risk reaping the bad with the good. If supernatural gods exist to help us, and we cannot empirically prove or disprove their existence but just *feel* it, why should not supernatural devils exist to plague us with bad things on earth and with a hellish existence (for eternity!) in our next life? The fact that so many religious people have created hells as well as heavens indicates that once we believe in the latter, we also can easily create the former. Is our hypoth-

esizing good deities worth the risks of our also hypothesizing bad ones and needlessly plaguing ourselves?

9. A moderate belief—for example, "Since gods are unlikely, I don't believe they exist"—acknowledges that since there is no evidence for gods, it can be *assumed* that there aren't any. A strong Belief—for example, "Since gods are very unlikely, I am damned sure that they don't exist!"—is a *pronounced* Belief, and therefore *is* emotional. Strong beliefs *imply* certainty, which is something of an emotional *prejudice*.

Noting the foregoing reasons for being wary of *feeling* that supernatural entities exist when we can't empirically prove or disprove them, how do I deal with my clients who insist that they do and that believing they do definitely helps them?

I merely say, first, "That's fine! If you think God or other unobservable things help you, by all means keep that belief. REBT holds that any positive belief can help you—and yours seems to do so. But don't forget that, in collaboration with God, you can also use the principles of REBT to considerably help yourself. Many people use REBT by itself to enhance their mental health and enjoyment. But you can use it with any of your religious philosophies to benefit yourself. If you want to teach your religious views to others, feel free to do so. But if you have any conflict between spiritual ideas and REBT, by all means tell me about it and let's resolve your conflict."

I also frequently show my clients what I point out in chapters 4 and 5—that many of the main REBT philosophies overlap with many religious ideas, and the two therefore reinforce each other. If my clients ask me directly what my religious attitudes are, I honestly and directly tell them and may discuss various issues without getting into any arguments. I also tell them that if they feel uncomfortable with a nonreligious person like myself, I can always help them to find a more religious therapist. I rarely have any trouble in this respect, although the great majority of my clients subscribe to some religion and often have firm and pronounced views that go with it.

I have more trouble with some of my clients who, I would say, religiously believe in psychoanalytic, Gestalt, or other kinds of therapy. If these views and practices seriously conflict with REBT principles, I show them what the conflict is and try to help them experiment with our methods, to discover how effective they are. If there is a serious clash, I again try to help them find a therapist with more compatible views.

Naturally, I lose some clients because of religious, spiritual, and other ideological differences. But as long as I give them unconditional other-acceptance and unconditional life-acceptance (or high frustration tolerance), we almost always get by without serious discord. Acceptance rather than heated argument does the trick!

Another important issue: A number of my clients can't tolerate other people's religious attitudes—including some of their relatives, friends, and business associates. In these cases, I encourage them to keep their own religious philosophies and even to hold them strongly if they will. But I show them that however "wrong," "stupid," or "harmful" others are religiously, their own upsetness about others' *ideas* arises from their damning of the others for their "horrible" religious attitudes. Damnation is fanaticism and bigotry.

By teaching UOA and ULA to religionists who won't tolerate differences with others, I have used REBT many times to reduce religious and antireligious prejudices and fighting. REBT opposes fanaticism of all kinds, especially that which leads to bickering and violence. Its "religion" is one of peace—of live and let live—of the reduction of bigotry and fanaticism.

8

Zen Buddhism and Rational Emotive Behavior Therapy

Rational Emotive Behavior Therapy has always been somewhat close to some main aspects of Buddhism and of Zen Buddhism. When I was giving up my practice of psychoanalysis, from 1953 onward, I explored what seemed to be more efficient techniques of therapy, reread many ancient and modern philosophers, and especially found helpful the ancient Greeks and Romans and the ancient Asians. I therefore incorporated much of the wisdom of Confucius, Lao-Tsu, and Gautama Buddha into REBT.

I soon became aware that there are many kinds of Buddhist groups and sects—and even several kinds of Zen Buddhists. So although I, like a number of other therapists, adopted several Zen theories and practices, I also modified or revised some of their teachings. But I kept some trenchant aspects of Zen.

For example, Buddhism is an active-directive practice and induces people to avoid pure theorizing about one's state and *do* something to change it. It *shows* its adherents what to do and *models* new behaviors. It uses relaxation and distraction techniques, especially various forms of meditation. It assumes that human life is "suffering" and difficult for all of us—but that we can successfully *accept* and *cope with* its hassles. It promotes "enlightenment" instead of, as Western civilization does, material accomplishment. It is very practical and down to earth. It de-emphasizes ego-aggrandizement and holier-than-thouness. It shows people that, when they make their wants and desires into *dire needs*, they become neurotic, and at times, this encourages them to attempt to reach the unusual state of desirelessness. It partially emphasizes self-actualization. It uses some metaphorical explanations of disturbance and health.

All Buddhism and all Zen are not alike, and some attitudes and practices are contradictory. But many bring at least palliative release from stress, strain, and suffering and may produce peace and harmony. Therefore, such therapists as Erich Fromm, Karen Horney, Alan Watts, and Paul Watzlawick often used them.

Maurits Kwee, who practices REBT as well as Arnold Lazarus's multimodal therapy, has particularly espoused Zen Buddhism. I wrote a paper with him, "The Interface between Rational Emotive Behavior Therapy (REBT) and Zen," in 1998. I think that he is a little too enthusiastic about Zen at times, but I shall include in this chapter some Buddhist views that we both tend to endorse and also some that are too extreme for my tastes.

REBT doesn't completely use the Zen techniques I described three paragraphs back. I at times use them selectively and don't take some of them, such as meditation, to extremes. Meditation of all kinds—and there are many kinds—often works. But meditation is often a distraction technique that enables you to think of something other than the thing you are depressed or panicked about.

Thus, I have found that if you are worried about going to sleep, your view, "I must fall asleep! I've got to go to sleep soon!" will actually *keep* you from sleeping. If, instead, you meditate and say, "Om, om, om!" or any other monotonous phrase to yourself, you will often quickly go to sleep. However, your *philosophy* that staying awake is *awful* and that you *must* beautifully solve your current problems will largely be sidetracked but not removed by meditation. Your worrisome *attitude* remains and preferably should be disputed and surrendered. Unless you modify your attitude to "It's *preferable* to fall asleep and be fresh for tomorrow. But it's not *necessary* to do so," you will not thoroughly change it. You have to *work* at reorganizing it cognitively, strongly (emotionally), and behaviorally in order to steadily change it.

Zen and other forms of meditation can be quite useful because they *temporarily* shunt away worry and awfulizing. But they can be easily taken to unproductive extremes and lead to unhealthy passivity and lack of creativity and enjoyment. I have seen a number of clients who have meditated for an hour or two a day for several years and are still very anxious.

Zen meditation may also be "thought stopping." You force yourself to watch your thoughts instead of evaluating how disruptive they are. That indeed interrupts and removes your *panicky* thoughts, which is helpful. But it doesn't automatically provide you with *constructive* thinking. Indeed, it may block the constructive thought, "If I don't obsess about not sleeping, I will probably fall asleep. But If I don't sleep, no catastrophe will ensue and I'll merely be tired tomorrow—but still get by." That constructive thought will not only help you sleep tonight but also stop your catastrophizing about sleep on other nights.

Zen is usually practical and doesn't bother about theoretical questions like, "Who created the universe?" and "Does God exist?" Fine! But meditation may passively discourage you from *action*, which involves (1) *thinking, planning, and scheming* to improve poor conditions; (2) *feeling* that what exists is often not desirable and working to change it; (3) and *doing* something about getting poor results and *actively trying* to improve them. Does it sound like meditating at length will help you in these respects?

When you think and think *too much* about failing to sleep or succeeding at a project or whether your beloved really cares for you, your obsessive panic blocks your goals. But if you meditate and distract yourself from obsessing, you may frequently go to the other extreme, think *too little* about your wishes and *not* try to have them fulfilled. Of course, that inactivity probably won't kill you, but neither will it fulfill you.

In the one life we'll ever have, most of us would like to have maximum self-actualization—meaning to try pathways we really might like but don't yet try. If we meditate *about* our wishes and nonwishes, we might truly discover what they are and more enjoy them. Lovely! But Zen meditation often seems to be the opposite of this kind of absorbing meditation. If anything, it often consists of forcing yourself to shunt away low frustration tolerance when you don't get what you really desire, but *also* to shunt away desire itself. This stops your *cultivating* your wishes, *broadening* their possibilities, and enjoying life *more*. In a dull, uninteresting world, this may protect you from whining about its restrictions. But in a world that has many potentially enjoyable pursuits, prolonged meditation may result in minimal self-actualization. Some therapists, such as Maurits Kwee, see Zen as releasing your freedom to be truly "yourself" and to therefore promote your self-actualizing. But are they realistically acknowledging the dulling and downing of self-fulfillment that easily goes with steady meditation?

All of which leads me to see that the Buddhist view that "life is suffering" may be true—but also prone to exaggeration. In Buddha's lifetime, some twenty-five hundred years ago, life was without many of our present conveniences—for example, without electricity and insect control—and therefore entailed, with few exceptions, more hassles and fewer joys. Minimizing people's suffering took precedence over maximizing their pleasures. Restrictive therapeutic methods like meditation often worked very well under these conditions. What did downtrodden people have to lose? Especially when Asian (and other) individuals had a short life span compared with people today. "A short life and a meditative one" may have been an excellent slogan for Buddha's day. But equally today?

By a similar token, few people in ancient days probably retired from work—or from taking care of their relatives—at an early age, and few lived for thirty or more
years on social security, investments, or other sinecures.
If they lived to a ripe old age, they were probably
affected by illness, poverty, and onerous labor. No
wonder that so many lives consisted of "suffering" and
therefore could well embrace distracting meditation as a
"wonderful" way out.

Meditation, particularly as it is often practiced in Zen,
is hardly for everyone. Those who regularly practice it
appear to be a select minority—such as wise men, monks,
acolytes, educated people, and others. Did the majority of
Buddhists really spend much time meditating? Do they
today still do so? I have some doubts about this. Perhaps
middle-class and well-to-do people often practiced Zen
meditation. But farmers, laborers, and members of lower
socioeconomic classes? Again, I have my serious doubts.

Let me again make an important point. If, as I have
been showing, some of the main philosophies of many
religious people overlap with those who hold a philosophy close to REBT, this agreement probably indicates that
these social and moral philosophies tend to work in practice. Fanatical religionists may use them differently from
moderate religionists and from people with little religion.
Many people may ostensibly subscribe to these practical
philosophies but actually follow much different rules. But
all over the world, some aspects of these attitudes seem
practical enough to at least be given lip service.

This hardly proves that humanist moral philosophies, such as those favored by REBT and by many religions, are perfectly "right" and "good" and will work out best for people most of the time. Humanism has its difficulties and failings. Like the American Bill of Rights, it *sounds* good to millions of us—but some of it may not be totally beneficial. Don't forget that what is called "good" and "bad" differs widely in various cultures and in the same culture at different times.

From this critique of Zen (and other) meditation, you may conclude that I find it pretty useless. But that's not true. I find it questionable as a comprehensive technique of Disputing irrational, self-defeating Beliefs—unless it is combined with some philosophy that more or less tackles those Beliefs.

Take, for example, the Zen technique that if you have panicky Beliefs—"I've got to complete this project very well or else I'm worthless!"—you can beneficially meditate. True. But you can also use REBT to directly Dispute your Beliefs by asking yourself, "How does this follow? Will failing this project really *make* me worthless?" The answer: "Obviously, it won't and can't. My *project* may turn out to be foolish and of no worth. But me, the doer of the project, totally worthless? Ridiculous! My conclusion doesn't follow from the fact that one of my *projects* may be of little value."

Instead of Disputing my Irrational Belief about the value of my project *equaling* the value of *me*, I may attempt to use the Zen technique of *observing* my thought—"The value of my project is the *same* as my value as a human." I meditate about it but do not assess it. But seeing it nonassessively *implies* that it is far-fetched and invalid. The only thing that *makes me* worthless for turning out a poor project *is* the *evaluation* of myself.

First, I evaluate the project as "poor," which may be correct, if others think so, too, or if the project comes to naught. Okay. But then I overgeneralizingly evaluate me, the doer of the project, as consequently being worthless. How does that second evaluation—of my total worth—follow from my (and other people's) assessment of the "goodness" of *me*, a whole *person*? It doesn't. For I do and can do many other projects than this one, and they may often be assessed as effective or "good" projects.

If, during meditation, I *only* assess my project as "good" or "bad" but *don't* assess my *personhood* the same way, this *implies* that I, myself, my being *is* unrateable and that my conclusion, "I am a bad person for turning out this execrable project," is also inaccurate.

My looking at my Irrational Belief, "I, like my project, am rateable," may therefore be a form of Disputing or invalidating it. It might lead to the same conclusion that Disputing of Irrational Beliefs generally does—that I am neither a good or a bad *person*—just a person who, this time, has produced a good or bad *project*. Correct! But while meditating, I can also look at but not evaluate my irrational conclusion—"My poor project *makes me* a worthless person"—and still fail to see that it is a false conclusion.

Assuming that most techniques of Zen meditation can work therapeutically, but not as elegantly as hard-headed Disputing of Irrational Beliefs, and assuming that they work palliatively and temporarily, why use them at all? The answer is: They work, and sometimes quickly work, for a chosen therapeutic purpose, and what works, works!

Take my own desire to fall asleep quickly at bedtime, which I prefer to do since lying awake takes time, interferes with my getting enough sleep, and makes me tired the next day. A waste! I have had this problem all my life and do much better conquering it with meditation than with other methods. I discovered that two main things keep me awake when I want to go to sleep: First, worry—about sleeping itself or about what unfortunate things *may* occur in my life and second, exciting thoughts, feelings, and actions.

As to the first problem, I conquered it almost fifty years ago when I created REBT and used it on myself. When attempting to sleep, I make myself *concerned* about various misfortunes that may (easily!) occur, but I fully realize that obsessively worrying and catastrophizing about them will, if anything, make them *more* likely to happen. So I sometimes plan what to do *if* they occur—and then I think about more pleasant things and put myself to sleep.

As for thinking about exciting things, I permit myself to do so for a while but then resort to meditation. I find that meditating on a mantra is monotonous and that monotony quickly puts me to sleep. So I monotonously say to myself, "Relax, relax, relax!" or "Sleep, sleep, sleep!" Almost always, I doze off in a few minutes. If I occasionally still have real difficulty, I *strongly* (emotionally) repeat "Relax, relax, relax" and force myself to use body motions—such as deep breathing—to accompany it.

I have used this relaxation meditation technique for years and frequently still do; I have taught it to many of my clients and friends. Although I am still hesitant about using complex meditation methods, like viewing my own thoughts but *not* evaluating them, I think that simple ones like monotonously relaxing work far better for quickly falling asleep. But they are not the best means for Disputing anxious, depressed, and angry thoughts and feelings. At least, not for me.

As Zen masters and some psychotherapists have found, there are many ways of teaching Zen practices effectively. Lectures and stories work, but so do metaphors, fables, and other literary devices, so I frequently use them. One of my favorite stories I took from a Zen parable:

> Two Zen monks, an old Master of ninety and a young novice of twenty, came to a flooded stream where a beautiful young woman of nineteen was waiting. "Masters," she said to both of them, "the stream is totally flooded and is very rough, and I can't swim. Will you please help me to get across it?" The young novice was shocked at this request, for he would have had to take this lovely young woman in his arms and carry her across the stream. "I am sworn to chastity," he said, "and unfortunately I cannot help you."
>
> The old master thought for a moment, then said, "You know, it's really against our rules, but I'll try to help you." So he lifted the woman in his arms, let her put her own arms around his neck, carried her, and put her down safely on the other side of the stream. She thanked him profusely, and the two Zen monks continued their journey. The young man was very troubled by what had

happened, and soon angrily burst out: "Master, how could you do a dreadful thing like that—take this beautiful young woman in your arms, let her put her lovely arms around your neck, her gorgeous breasts pressing against your breast, and *carry* her like that across the stream?" "My son," the old master quietly replied, *"you're still carrying her."*

Most of my clients and friends quickly grasp this metaphor and learn a useful Zen lesson from it.

Zen specializes in paradoxical thinking, because life *is* paradoxical, and seeing it that way increases your understanding. But many of Zen's paradoxical sayings seem to be *too* clever. They make you think and rarely give practical solutions to problems but instead "profound" contradictory ones.

D. T. Suzuki tells us that "Carry away the farmer's oxen and make off with the hungry man's food" is a favorite phrase with the Zen masters, who think we can best cultivate the spiritual life of farmers and fill their souls hungry for the substance of things. In REBT terms, however, how does this paradox explain (1) what *is* the substance of *things*? (2) How will acting paradoxically fill up your hungry soul? (3) How will it help the farmer or the hungry man? (4) If you *now* see that helping the farmer and the hungry man is a conventional plan that paradoxically will lead you nowhere, how will it show you how to choose an unconventional better life? Clever and unusual instructions, but where do they lead? What do you do with your "hungry soul" when you antagonize the farmer and the hungry man? Especially if nonparadoxically they kill you?

In addition to paradox, Suzuki describes several other verbal methods and one direct experiential method of arriving at Zen understanding. The verbal methods are (1) the denial of opposites, (2) contradiction—the Zen master's negation of what he himself has stated; (3) the affirmation of irrational Zen ways of looking at things; (4) repetition, and even parrotlike repetition, of what the masters have said; (5) and making an exclamatory utterance in response to a question instead of giving an intelligible answer.

Suzuki gives many examples of how these verbal Zen methods worked to convince questioners of the "truth" of Zen. I read all of them carefully but was not in the least convinced that the specific answers of the masters *really* worked. These masters *reported* that all five verbal responses convinced their questioners, but that hardly proved that any or all of them were in themselves effective.

Looking a little further and "deeper," I think I discovered *why* these verbal techniques "convinced" the novices of Zen "truths." When the masters used one of these "surefire" methods—repetition of what they heard and sometimes "parrot-like repetition"—they were thoroughly convincing because, Suzuki writes, "The words themselves are mere sounds, and the inner sense is to be read in the repetition itself if anywhere. The understanding must come from one's inner life."

Ah! That's it. The understanding of Zen doesn't follow from anything the master does or says but "from one's [that is, the questioner's] inner life." It comes from the intuitive experience of the student, *not* from the paradoxical remarks of the teacher.

A little later on, in explaining the nonverbal or "the direct method" by which a master teaches the novice how to understand and use Zen, Suzuki says: "The truth of Zen is the truth of life, and life means to live, to move, to act, not merely to reflect." And again: "There is something stronger than ratiocination. We may call it will, or instinct, or more comprehensively, will. Where this will acts, there is Zen."

Ah, again. The student of Zen does not *reflect* on what the master says (or doesn't say). He listens with his will, his intuition, his own experiencing. And he *acts* and *lives* by will, intuition, and personal experience. So he *brings* himself and his intuition to the master, and therefore he innately *understands* and *lives* Zen—even if he had no master. The master *reminds* him of his own inner strength and self-discipline, which he intuitively acts upon.

As for me, I am not ready to receive any master's verbal answers—because, I would guess, I am "naturally" more logical than intuitive. My innate logic easily wins out over my intuition. So all of Suzuki's verbal techniques of imparting Zen do not convince me. By direct action and will maybe I *almost* reach Zen, but supposedly my logic and rationality keep getting in my way. I am not intuitively and semimystically *ready* for Zen, so, at most, I have glimpses of it.

"When I have raised the hand, there is Zen," says Suzuki. "But when I assert that I have raised the hand, Zen is no more." Intuition, mysticism, and direct movement disappear, and I am left with consciousness and thinking—which won't miraculously work.

If I am correct about Suzuki and his citing of Zen masters who "answered" their questioners, what I have been saying in this chapter is (paradoxically?) useful and not so useful. Many of Zen's slogans and techniques are cognitive-behavioral. They are similar to REBT or variations of it that can be integrated with it and effectively used—at least with some people some of the time. So I use them.

Zen still includes, however, a semimystical, intuitive, personal experiencing set of core beliefs and practices that do not fit in with empirical and scientific "prejudices" and that can be taught only to people who already, with their own intuitive biases, resonate to it. Suzuki claims that Zen is different from other mystical general statements concerning God or the world because it "carries its paradoxical assertions into every detail of our life." In some ways it does. But it often still holds on to many of the same kind of antifactual propositions of other unprovable and undisprovable "explanations" of other mystical creeds. Moral: follow and use it with caution! It may easily give you paradoxical and far from practical answers.

This chapter is by no means a comprehensive critique of Zen Buddhism, but let me discuss two more of its important concepts. First, "no-thought." Zen believers, as Emmanuel Berger puts it, are overwhelmingly intuitive. They indirectly perceive "the deeper meanings and possibilities inherent in things." They, as Allan Watts interprets, allow "the mind to operate on its own without attempting at the same time to observe, check, and control our thinking in order to achieve some intended effect." As I noted earlier, the students of the Zen masters presumably excel in intuitively grasping what the Zen masters are saying—or are not saying!

Zen practitioners who participate in athletic activities, such as swordsmanship, use spontaneous "no-thought" to supposedly allow their bodies, without giving *thought* to technique and without intellection, to respond intuitively and spontaneously to whatever occurs in their athletic contests. Without *trying* to get certain results, and thus dualistically making their thought its own object, they somehow— I say magically—get great results by exerting "no-thought."

Nice work, if you can do it! But in more behavioral terms, I hypothesize that Zen swordsmen and other "no-thought" athletes, after much *conscious* practice, ultimately learn to use their unconscious habits to work effectively. You do this same thing when you "automatically" drive your car while talking to a friend. You are not paying close attention to your driving, as you may be to your friend's conversation, but you really are *habitually* doing so. Your "no-thought" driving really has much thought—and especially practice—behind it. Zen Buddhist "no-thought," I guess, is mainly a different kind of thinking, but it really is not, as Zen theory implies, no thinking at *all*. It is made by Zen devotees to *appear* to be magical thoughtlessness in order to give special credit to the human ability to do two different things at once and have only *low-level* consciousness of doing one of them.

One additional point: If you try to *control* and get better results from your unconscious, habituated thinking, you often screw up and get worse results. You become self-conscious about your lack of self-consciousness and think that you *have to* know it works. Your franticness may then interfere with your more calmly investigating your "no-thought" to see if it really has some kind of thinking and planning included in it. Which it semiconsciously does!

Writers on Zen are fond of pointing out that your thinking about your thinking is too unspontaneous and unintuitive—and therefore ruins your hard-won freedom from intellectualizing. It is presumably anti-Zen. Devotees of Zen, because they don't fully analyze their thinking about thinking, miss the boat here.

If you carefully analyze your thinking, you often help yourself improve it—and make yourself *more* rational and effective. But, first, you had better not analyze it *while* you are doing it. That, as I have said, leads to confusion. If you try to see *how* you are hitting a tennis ball *while* you are hitting it as best you can, you are trying to have *two* thoughts *at once* and that often won't work. Preferably, you can think about *how* you hit the ball (well or badly) *later*—and you can even make videotapes of your playing to analyze later.

Let me see if I can make this clearer. You hit the tennis ball to your opponent's left side because you think he won't reach it and won't be able to retrieve it. But he does return it and you lose the point. You see that this is so and say to yourself, "Well, I won't try that again!" So you think about your thinking and the action that went with it, you revise your strategy, and you benefit from your thinking about your thinking.

If, however, as soon as you first think that you'd better hit the tennis ball to your opponent's left side, you simultaneously think, "No, he probably can return it from there, so

I'd better think, 'Maybe that's the wrong move. I'd better try his right side. Then maybe he'll return it badly and I'll win that point.'" You then have *two* thoughts, "I'd better hit it to his left side," *and* "No, I'd better hit it to his right side." These two thoughts clash and you hardly know *what* to do.

What I'm saying is that sometimes your corrective thinking about what you have thought and done is very useful if done at the proper time. But sometimes, if your second thought follows your first thought too quickly, you confuse yourself.

Also, if you think about your thinking *after* you've done it and got poor results but don't think about it *at the same time* you are doing it, you may benefit from doing so. Moreover, you had better watch your *musts* and *have to*s when you think about your thinking. Don't tell yourself, "I *must* see what I'm thinking! I *have to* improve my thinking!" *Prefer* to observe your thinking and to correct it if it is ineffective. Necessitizing about observing it and changing it will make you obsessively-compulsively *worry* about it. No go!

With "no-thought," then, and with "No thinking about my thinking!" you may help yourself be more spontaneous but can easily go to extremes and sneak in the *musts* you are trying to reduce. "No-thought" *may* have some good uses. But watch its extremes!

How about the Zen Buddhist concept of desirelessness or nirvana? Buddhism at times clearly seems to see that your goal or desire dualistically interacts with wanting to "conquer" your life and your environment and to thereby obtain what your *ego* or self wants. Both Zen and REBT say that this is *risky* because desires or preferences add to your life, but your direly *needing and demanding* that you get what you want and don't get what you don't want can easily get you into trouble—that is, *overly* frustrated, angry, and depressed. REBT endorses your preferences and encourages you to go for them, explore them, and soon enough experimentally change them and choose more realistic desires and avoidances. In fact, REBT says that you can actualize yourself and discover "who you (at this moment) are" by exploring many kinds of conventional (culture-favored) *and* unconventional enjoyments to see which work (and don't work) for you and your loved ones. *Guessing* what you may like and dislike and *trying out* these possibilities is perhaps the main way you can discover "yourself" and increase your self-actualization—as long as you don't turn your goals and desires into *dire needs*.

Buddhism agrees with REBT that *needs* are different from *desires*, especially since our environment has many *restrictions and barriers*. Buddhism's First Noble Truth, therefore, is that our mind doesn't fully grasp our dual subject-object relationships and has a biased or ignorant perception of unlimited reality (because we *desire* something, it *should* exist for us). We see the world as *static* instead of *free*, not as (it is) divided into discrete and limited classes. Our mind's conception of life is therefore an illusion (or *maya*) and is not really the way life *is*. As I noted before, Zen's First Noble Truth says that real life—and not what we see it as—is *suffering*. All of us have restriction of our desires and frustration about this restriction. We just cannot experience perfect pleasure or fulfillment of our desires. We are easily *deluded* that we can have eternal bliss. But we can't.

Following our perception of this illusion comes the Second Noble Truth of Buddhism. Desire consists of your constantly viewing the forms of reality into discrete categories created by your mind and *is* a false sense of self. You view conditions as constant when they are really transient or evolving and you thus trap yourself with perceptual frustration or *samsara,* the round of birth and death—a state of dualistic or constricted biased apperception, as James Croake and Ronald Rusk call it. You thereby try to maintain a (false) state of uniqueness and individual superiority (as Alfred Adler noted) instead of the healthy *un*dualistic state of social interest, community interest, and communal intuition—which would help you to see your and others' life as it *is* and to solve your self-in-your-community problem.

The Buddhist solution of your giving up your false sense of environment and self-duality and making yourself separate from your "superiority" to others is nirvana. You achieve this state—Buddha's Third Noble Truth—by surrendering the false notion of your self being separate from your environment and from others by obtaining Enlightenment or Buddhahood or nirvana. You then give up the illusion (*maya*) of having a separate self, lose self-concern for individual uniqueness, and embrace the Fourth Noble Truth, which, say Croake and Rusk, "prescribes the means to end all suffering. You then take the Eightfold Path, which leads to Nirvana."

This combining of Adler's *social interest* with Buddhist selflessness or nirvana seems to make much sense. Both these "enlightened" philosophies of life say that you (and other people) delude yourself by seeing your individual "selfish" self as dualistically *separate* from your environment when, actually, the two are coalesced into *one* unified life. This illusion makes for confusion and misery, which you can escape by embracing monolithic reality and totally *accepting* your individual life goals and your inevitable *connection* with the *oneness* of you *in* the universe and *with* the community of the world. Using the four Noble Truths of Buddhism, you do this by ridding yourself of your illusions (*karma*) and your neurotic strivings for personal "success" that produce one-sided life goals.

By giving up *mere* personal desire and by desperately trying to maintain a *separate* sense of self even though my self *includes* and cannot be separated from my *interactions* with my being in the environment and being integrally related to other people in my community, I achieve selflessness or nirvana. I do this by meditation (which shows me that I can stop *clinging to* and *needing* the fulfillment of my individual desires), by focusing on community or social interest, and by intuitively sensing and experiencing my self at one *with* the world instead of separate from it.

Now this Buddhist conception of how I (and other humans) have dualistic illusions (*maya*) about my (and other people's) life in the environment of the world seems to be at least partially accurate and overlaps with the theories of REBT—to some extent. REBT holds that (1) you are restricted and frustrated by your environment and your desires *not* to be restricted but to (almost perfectly) fulfill your pleasure-seeking urges; (2) you are frequently deluded that you *can* unrestrictedly fulfill your desires and goals; (3) you keep encountering harsh suffering that shows you that full freedom to get what you want does not *exist;* (4) you nevertheless egoistically decide that you not only *preferably* should fulfill your desires but that because you have them, you *must* fulfill them; (5) you unrealistically often see yourself as a *special person* and as *better than other people;* (6) you foolishly denigrate your entire being, your *self,* when you see that your illusion of grandiosity or specialness does not hold up; (7) your dualistic and contradictory illusions about you and other people almost inevitably—*because* they are false and your limitations are real—get you into neurotic *dis*illusionment and depression; (8) you see no way out of these dilemmas—as there *should* be! So you make yourself more disturbed—and, often, disturbed about *feeling* disturbed and encountering even more frustrations about your desires and your restrictions.

A pretty pickle! REBT helps you resolve it—but not completely—by tackling your unrealistic illusions (*maya*) and fully *accepting* your own limitations, other people's frustrating you, and the world's limitations that you try to improve but that you can't for the present change. The philosophy and practice of REBT enables you to feel *healthily* sorry, regretful, and disappointed instead of *unhealthfully* angry, depressed, and self-deprecating when you strive for what you desire but do not quickly get it. It teaches you to realistically—without illusion—change the restrictions that you *can* change, to *accept* those that you cannot change, and as Reinhold Niebuhr said, to have the wisdom to see the difference!

Zen Buddhism resembles REBT in that it helps you dispel some of your important illusions and presumably accept the "reality" of your life and yourself. It also shows you that you and your individual self are not the center of the universe and in its own way it helps you give up rating yourself as a good or a bad *person*. In this respect, it agrees with Alfred Korzybski and with REBT. Self-rating, according to Zen, separates you from your oneness with the universe.

Unfortunately, Zen's nirvana not only gives up your individual uniqueness but also implies that it doesn't really exist. You have no *self* and had better not pretend that you do. You have only oneness with the universe.

This seems to be a gross exaggeration. First, you do have an individual *self* or *personality*. You are not *just* the universe, although you are *part* of it. You *are* different from all other people—at least, in some respects. When you die, you don't exist anymore—although the universe in which you live will exist. It doesn't any longer exist for *you*—but it does exist for other (live) people.

So *some* unity exists, since while you live you always live in connection with your environment. You need it and *relate* to it and to other people. But to say that you exist in and with your environment hardly denies that there is, for a while at least, an individual and personal person call you. To a considerable extent, a dualism does exist—you are you *and* are your environment. After you are gone, the world will exist (1) for others and (2) by itself. It won't evaporate!

Because of your unique heredity and the social environment that is always an intrinsic *part* of your life, you have both individual and social desires and preferences. No one else seems to have all your individual goals and desires—since you are different from all other people in having some unique desires and in their *developing* and *changing*. Your social desires are *somewhat* community learned, but even they are partially different from other people's social proclivities and actions. Again, you are still you—with both individual *and* social unique aspects.

To reach this new state of nirvana, as Croake and Rusk point out, you would have to achieve "annihilation of desire; not the loss of awareness, but the loss of self-concern for individual uniqueness."

Just try! As long as you are aware—that is, conscious that you are you—desire is innate and not merely learned. It appears to be a biological (and social) *given*. Unless you distinctly desire to continue living, moving, eating, loving, lusting, perceiving, thinking, feeling, and behaving, how can you survive in any environment? Again, just try it and see!

Even desires that you partially learn—such as to drink milk or to get along with other people—you become accustomed to and desire—yes, desire—to keep going. If not, how can you survive?

You are born and raised with awareness *and* desire. They both have their disadvantages. You can have false awareness—be aware of nonexistent dangers. You can desire many harmful things, like too much heat or freezing cold, like malnutritious food or drug addictions. You can change your desires—curb or increase them. But can you make yourself truly desireless—and still survive very long? I doubt it!

Where will extreme nirvana really get you? Pretty dead. Taken to extremes, to be self-aware but deny all the desires that you have in your awareness, is to be blah—alive but not for very long! REBT tries to keep you very much alive—and kicking. Some aspects of Zen Buddhism may also help. But extremist Zen? I wonder.

9

The Social Philosophy of Rational Emotive Behavior Therapy

Practically all people, whether they are aware of it or not, have a political, economic, and social philosophy about which they think, feel, and act. Politically, they are usually liberal, conservative, or revolutionary. Economically, they are often capitalistic or collectivistic. Socially, they are quite interested in other people or little interested; they also are actively engaged with their community or pretty much disengaged from it. I have written about REBT's philosophy in regard to social, political, and economic affairs in several articles and books, and in this chapter I shall summarize some of my main views on its social attitudes.

In particular, REBT includes a clear-cut philosophy of social involvement, morality, and community responsibility. While it stresses unconditional self-acceptance and favors enlightened self-interest, it also emphasizes that people live in families and social groups. If people do not have considerable social interest, they will fight with others, lose support, help sabotage their group, and interfere with their own well-being and happiness. As Alfred Adler said, social interest and individual interest promote human survival.

Consequently, REBT encourages its clients and other people to work at having unconditional other-acceptance. If they think, feel, and behave cooperatively and responsibly and help other people's interests along with their own, REBT assumes that both they and others will be much less angry and the world much better.

In my writings and talks for the past twenty years, I have especially pointed out that modern technology has provided hostile and bigoted people—such as suicide bombers—with the most deadly weapons and will eventually, if it keeps advancing, enable them to manufacture atomic bombs in their kitchens or bathrooms. Then the fanatically hostile people—who now number millions of rabid haters—will be able perhaps to wipe out all of us. Not today yet—but maybe within a few more decades.

Unconditional other-acceptance, if ever achieved by practically everyone, is perhaps the only philosophy that will save us from mass destruction. It requires, however, long-term education of children, adolescents, and adults— not merely, as now, therapeutically given to disturbed people, as in REBT and a few kinds of forgiveness therapy, but to everyone who may turn into a dangerous killer.

Till that time, UOA can be something of an experiment in saving the world. If it can be shown that REBT and other fully accepting therapies can help disturbed people turn away from psychopathic hating, then it may be possible to teach the rest of the world UOA.

Right after the September 11, 2001, terrorist attacks, I was asked a question on the REBT Web site about dealing with terrorism. I immediately answered this question:

How would one go about using REBT in order to cope and to help others cope with the tragic events that took place on September 11? I am looking for a proactive way to deal with the brutality of this act, but find that my Irrational Beliefs and *should*s are getting in my way. I replied:

My (and your) Irrational Beliefs and *should*s that get in our way of sensibly dealing with terrorism probably include:

1. "I absolutely *must* be able to figure out a way to stop terrorists from acting so brutally and killing and maiming so many people, and there is something very weak and inadequate about me because I can't find a way to stop this kind of terrorism."
2. "The terrorists and their backers have perpetrated some of the worst deeds imaginable; this makes them *completely rotten people* who *should absolutely be exterminated*—quickly—since only killing all of them will stop this deed from happening again."
3. "Because the world is so full of cruel violence and terrorism, it is a totally despicable place and I cannot continue to live in it and be at all happy."

These ideas are irrational because, as Alfred Korzybski noted in *Science and Sanity* in 1933, they are unrealistic and illogical overgeneralizations that render people "unsane." My 1962 book, *Reason and Emotion in Psychotherapy*, showed that all three of these beliefs— and many similar absolutistic *should*s and *must*s—lead you (and innumerable other people) to make yourself not only very sad and displeased with the terrorists' abominable behavior, but also to dysfunctionally overwhelm yourself with panic, rage, and depression. Thus, the first of these Irrational Beliefs will cause you to loathe your entire self, or personhood, not to only deplore your weakness and inadequacy to halt terrorism. The second of these Irrational Beliefs will make you thoroughly despise the terrorists (and all other people who do cruel deeds) and consume yourself with rage. The third of these Irrational Beliefs will make you hopelessly depressed about the present and future state of the world and encourage you to obsessively contemplate—and perhaps actually commit—suicide.

Ironically, these three self-defeating *should*s and *must*s are probably very similar to those held by the terrorists, who unsanely killed themselves and thousands of innocent people for what they considered a holy crusade. They first considered themselves powerless because they could not stop America from "cruelly" siding with their enemies; and they therefore felt that they *absolutely had* to punish America to prove that they themselves were powerful and worthwhile individuals. Second, they devoutly believed that Americans *absolutely must not* oppose their position and that *all Americans are complete devils* who deserve to be wiped out. Third, they dogmatically convinced themselves there is no use living in and trying to lead a happy life in such a totally evil world; and therefore, by killing the infidels, they would attain eternal, blissful life. So, with these unsane beliefs, they enthusiastically killed themselves along with many innocent people.

If you and the rest of America and world citizens keep reinforcing your Irrational Beliefs, you will enrage yourself against the terrorists and their backers and in the process will likely encourage them to increase their fury against Americans and other people who oppose them; and you will encourage more retaliation by them, by us again, until the cycle of retaliation precipitates a worldwide war and quite possibly the end of our planet. As ancient lore and modern history have amply shown, love begets love and hatred and violence beget increased hatred and violence—with no end in sight!

You ask how REBT would help you cope with and help others cope with the tragic events of September 11, 2001. That requires a long answer, which I can only briefly summarize here.

First, you can use rational emotive behavior therapy (REBT) to teach yourself—and others—*unconditional self-acceptance*. That is, you fully accept yourself with all your warts and flaws, while heartily disliking and doing your best to change some of your self-defeating behaviors and destructive actions toward others.

Second, you can use REBT to *unconditionally accept all other people* as persons, no matter how abominably they act. You can, of course, firmly try to induce them, in a variety of ways, to change their self-sabotaging and immoral thoughts, feelings, and actions. In Christian terms, you unconditionally accept all *sinners* but not their *sins*. Ultimately some behaviors may require sanctions or imprisonment for individuals.

Third, you can *unconditionally accept life*, with its immense problems and difficulties, and teach yourself to have high frustration tolerance. As Reinhold Niebuhr said, you strive to change the unfortunate things you can change, to accept (but not to like) those that you cannot change, and to have the wisdom to know the difference.

If you achieve a good measure of these three REBT philosophies—that is, unconditional self-acceptance, unconditional other-acceptance, and unconditional life-acceptance—will you therefore be able to convince terrorists to change their absolutistic bigoted ways? Not exactly. But you will cope much better with terrorism, help others to cope with it, and model behavior that can, if you strongly encourage it to be followed around the world, eventually reduce it to a minimum. This will take many years to effect, and will require immense and persistent educational efforts by you and others to promote peaceful and cooperative solutions instead of hateful and destructive "solutions" to serious national and international difficulties. If we fail to work on our own belief systems to produce this long-term purpose, we will only ensure renewed terrorism for decades, and perhaps centuries, to come.

Are you willing to keep relentlessly working for REBT's recommendations for self-peace, peace to other humans, and peace to the world? If so, you may help people of goodwill to think, plan, and execute eventual answers to terrorism and many other serious world problems.

My answer to how we can deal with fanatical political and religious international hatred and terrorism may seem too Pollyannaish. Before we can implement any widespread educational plan against this great danger, it may be too late, and suicidal squads may already be planning a worldwide nuclear holocaust that would wipe out themselves and most of the rest of us. But if we continue to war against actual and potential terrorists, and if our warring "prophylactic" actions continue to engender suicidal reprisals, what other plans do we have to eventually educate all humanity against continued terrorism? Who has a better answer to that question than worldwide teachers of unconditional other-acceptance?

My writings against fanatical bigotry and intolerance in the realm of politics and economics began in the 1930s when I was, first, a politico-economic and antifascist revolutionist. This was before I originated REBT, so I still evaluated people, and not merely their deeds, as "bad people" and "villains" who we revolutionists would "legitimately" damn and kill. If I and my fellow revolutionists could conquer and annihilate Hitler and Stalin and their supporters, I would have been happy with those results. In other words, I was an extreme and fanatical politico-economic revolutionist, and I even read some materials on manufacturing bombs and other weapons and how to deal with our (the revolutionists') opponents if they violently tried to stop our "noble" efforts to overthrow the reactionary order and replace it with a new one.

This was quite the opposite of unconditional other-acceptance, to say the least! But I gave up this fanatical revolutionary attitude when I saw that it didn't exactly work, that it had some utopian aspects, and that Hitler and Stalin were not going to be overthrown by a small band of ardent revolutionists such as the group with which I was affiliated (New America).

I also saw that a number of revolutionists and fellow travelers were working for the politico-economic changing of the oppressive systems that existed, but few were really working to bring about a highly desirable sex revolution. I had seen this from my adolescent years onward and often got my associates to agree with me that our society was much too sexually restricted. But now that I was giving up the cause of political revolution, I decided to devote myself to helping promulgate a sex revolution in the United States and Western civilization. Though I disliked sexual puritans and reactionaries, I didn't exactly hate them and want to annihilate them. I would work for the sex revolution only with words and certainly not with violent acts.

Along with working for the sex revolution, I also, somewhat later, began to be a psychotherapist—and then, as is my reforming nature, I first attempted to change psychoanalysis and make it more scientific. So I wrote several articles and a monograph, *An Introduction to the Scientific Principles of Psychoanalysis*. Although my monograph was widely quoted by scientifically oriented writers who already were skeptical of psychodynamic theories and their therapeutic effectiveness, it convinced virtually no hard-wired analysts to change their methods. I decided that my cause was pretty hopeless and started to think about substituting a better system or therapy—namely, Rational Emotive Behavior Therapy—for the liberal form of psychoanalysis that I was practicing in the early 1950s. I also continued my revolutionary sex writings, especially with my 1951 book, *The Folklore of Sex*; my 1953 book, *Sex, Society, and the Individual*; and my 1954 book, *The American Sexual Tragedy*. These led a little later to *Sex without Guilt* in 1958, *The Art and Science of Love* in 1960, and then several best-selling sex-love books in the 1960s.

Because my books on sex, especially *The Art and Science of Love*, were mainly written after I had created REBT, they combined my revolutionary views on sex with this new form of therapy. In the 1960s, I therefore became a double revolutionary in the field of psychotherapy and sex. Both fields made me notorious and criticizable. Many therapists wouldn't accept REBT because I was "too controversial" in the sex area, and many people wouldn't accept my sex and love views because I was "too controversial" in the psychotherapy field. But because I had been a politico-economic rebel and a declared atheist from age twelve onward, I was not disturbed about the criticism I received for my sex and therapy minority views. If anything, I liked the challenge of distinctly disagreeing with conventional attitudes and of not upsetting myself when most people were shocked by my unconventional ones. I find it challenging to take a lot of flak when my ways are quite different from others I encounter and *not* to make myself angry, anxious, or depressed about their negative views of me.

REBT has several main aspects to its social and relationship philosophy. The first is UOA. This is emphasized because, as I have been saying since I first created REBT, you are a unique individual who innately and by environmental teaching strongly desires to survive and be happy in the one life you'll most likely ever have. You can't live forever, but while you're alive your main goal is to continue living and have minimal pain and misery.

At the same time, you normally are a social creature who strives for help, support, approval, caring, relating, and loving. You like and benefit from this kind of activity, so you try to get along with and be reasonably close to others—not push them away or antagonize them. You observe their actions and their reactions to you and you try to have amicable and cooperative relationships with your family members, neighbors, and associates to protect yourself and enjoy your human contacts. You adopt practical attitudes toward and actions with other people. You *work* at achieving good social relations, sometimes with counseling and therapy.

Unconditional other-acceptance, therefore, recognizes your similarities and differences with others and tries to adjust serious differences and to arrange mutual interests with them. You observe others, try to cooperate with them, and sometimes try to get close to them. Your goal is to please others, and empathically to try to help them live and enjoy life, too. You socially *care*.

UOA, therefore, first enables you to understand and get along with others—and especially with significant others. Alfred Adler called it social interest, indicated how important it is for survival and happy living, and developed (along with other therapists) techniques for achieving it. Many ancient and modern philosophers also urge you to have considerable social interest.

REBT's philosophy of unconditional other-acceptance goes even further. As noted earlier, it not only teaches you the personal and community advantages of social interest, but also indicates its survival value today. First, it may protect you and your community from a destructive and warring life. Second, it may be practically the only way to stop fanatically angry people (including reckless and semipsychotic ones) from using increasingly destructive weapons to kill you, themselves, and practically everyone.

Here REBT has something important to say. It is not merely the existence of deadly weapons that endangers you and the rest of the world; it is that fact *plus* some people's fanatical urges to use these weapons. After all, nuclear fission and atomic bombs have been around since the early 1900s and several governments, including our own, can pulverize hoards of their enemies with them. But the people who control these governments are sane enough to use atomic power only once in a while because they fully realize it could destroy their enemies—and themselves. Once one country releases even a little of it, the repercussions can lead to a worldwide holocaust. But so far, we and other possessors of atomic power carefully keep it in check. We keep developing it and threatening to sometime use it. But we haven't implemented our threats *yet*.

Fanatically angry people are relatively few—but, as the events of the last several years show, they do exist and do create havoc. Will they continue to do so? Very likely! Will they, in extreme cases, construct atomic weapons and, without too much hesitation, actually use them? Again, quite likely! Conclusion: What can we do to head off these possible disasters?

As I said earlier, one answer is to teach everyone in the world—including fanatically disturbed people—social interest and unconditional other-acceptance. Everyone? Yes, eventually everyone. If even a few people resist this teaching and remain fanatically hostile, and if they are able to manufacture atomic warheads—poof, we're in trouble.

I may, of course, be too alarmist. Producing atomic weapons may always be too expensive for a minority of semipsychotic individuals to make and to use. Or other safeguards against their use may be invented. Very fine! But the real danger of atomic holocausts still exists. How are we going to use REBT's espousal to ward them off? How?

10

The Political and Economic Philosophy of Rational Emotive Behavior Therapy

Practically every social philosophy that people subscribe to includes and implies a political and economic philosophy, for all of us reside in a region or state that follows some set of rules and is rarely anarchic. It normally is democratic, liberal, or monarchical, dictatorial, or some combination of these systems. Economically, it is generally collectivist, capitalistic, or again partially both. Rarely is it absolutely one-sided, since dictatorships allow some liberal and democratic leeway, and collectivist communities (as in the Soviet Union) allow some private enterprise.

As I have mentioned before, I was in my youth a political revolutionist who wanted to overthrow dictatorships like Nazi Germany, Fascist Italy, and the dictatorship of Russia. At the same time, my ultimate goal was to have the state wither away or become unusually democratic. Though I also favored collectivism, I was not opposed to some amount of individualism and private enterprise. I was not very absolutistic or rigid in my politico-economic philosophy. I was ultimately liberal.

When I originated REBT, I was no longer a political revolutionary and was still a sexual revolutionist. That meant that I was exceptionally permissive and unconventional and believed that consenting adults were permitted to run their own sex lives as long as they did not take advantage of minors or disabled people and as long as they did not impose on or harm others. Pretty permissive!—and definitely liberal, democratic, and unconventional.

So with REBT. It holds that people who live in social groups—as practically all humans do—require rules, morals, and laws to enable them to live peacefully and safely. They can—and do—differ from each other and from other groups in many ways. But they normally had better refrain from assault, murder, stealing, kidnapping, and other acts that distinctly harm other people and are regularly banned and penalized. REBT generally agrees with regular moral rules because it is humanistic and opposes antihumanistic behaviors. It is hardly unique in this respect.

I read Ayn Rand's *The Fountainhead* when I was thirty-five years old and was new to the practice of psychotherapy. I thought that the book made a good case for individualism—but took it to somewhat fanatical extremes. Nor was I greatly opposed to her deification of capitalism although I thought that it, too, was exceptionally one-sided. By this time I had given up my own firm collectivist views, but I realized that the rabid capitalism that Rand fought for never had existed (as she admitted) because even capitalists controlled it to some degree and actually espoused considerable statism—at which Rand was horrified. *Pure* capitalism was contaminated by the controls that she violently opposed. Her *Fountainhead* hero, Howard Roark, was a fanatical freedom lover—and he destroyed his own architectural masterpiece when his enemies tried to (quite unethically!) restrict his sacred project. I could empathize with his resolutely fighting them—but not with his fanatical self-destructiveness. In some ways, I could see, he anticipated the suicide bombers who destroy both their enemies and themselves. Pretty crazy.

As Ayn Rand went on (for many years) to write *Atlas Shrugged* and other works with an obsessive-compulsive frenzy that savagely beat the drums for unalloyed superlibertarian views, she was frantically joined by a young psychologist who doted on her and her sacred writings, Nathaniel Branden, who formed the Nathaniel Branden Institute, which widely taught Rand's philosophy of objectivism. Branden, in turn, converted two of my psychologist friends, Roger Callahan and Lee Shulman, to fervent objectivism and came to see me to try to convert me, too. He at first claimed that objectivism was very similar to REBT, but I strongly disagreed.

After I read *Atlas Shrugged*, which Branden, Callahan, and Shulman thought was by far the greatest novel—not to mention politico-social text—ever written, I became an anti-Randist. I could plainly see that her one-track mind and feelings were as bigoted and absolutistic as those of Hitler and Stalin and that Branden was just as hooked on fanatical objectivism as Rand was.

Branden still thought he would win me over and make

REBT a vassal of objectivism. He even recommended me as a therapist to several students of the Branden Institute. I saw about a dozen of them for a while and found them all to be sacredizers of Rand, Branden, and objectivism. Rational they were not!

I decided to disassociate myself completely from practically all Rand's philosophies and tried to arrange a debate with her to make sure that no one would confuse our views and think that they could solve their emotional problems with objectivism *and* REBT. As far as I could see, the more they swore by objectivism, the more disturbed they would be.

Ayn Rand refused to debate with me (and other disagreers) because she always had to have the *only* and *final* word when she spoke. No interruptions. So I agreed to debate with Branden on the topic "Rational Emotive Psychotherapy versus Objectivist Psychology" and to have the debate organized by the Nathaniel Branden Institute and the Albert Ellis Institute (which was then called the Institute for Rational Living). It took place in 1968 at the old New Yorker Hotel and attracted eleven hundred people, only 10 percent of them favoring REBT and 90 percent favoring objectivism. Although I predicted that the Randians in the audience would be hostile to me and worshipping of Branden and Rand, I was shocked by their bigoted behavior. Every time I made a point for REBT and against objectivism, they let out boos and catcalls; every time Branden criticized me and REBT, they wildly cheered. The REBTers and the neutral people in the audience, on the other hand, politely applauded my points and clearly disagreed with Branden's barbs against me. As many of them reported later, they were shocked by Branden's vitriolic remarks and by the violent support of his followers.

I thought that I had done an adequate job of showing the basic differences between REBT and objectivism and tried to get our two institutes to publish the recording that was made of the debate so that it would have wide distribution. But Branden angrily refused to let it be published and gave no good reason for his refusal. He continued to be furious against me for the next thirty years; neither he nor Barbara Branden gave honest versions of our debate in their autobiographies.

To make matters much worse, Ayn Rand attended the debate as Branden's guest and had a screaming fit when I criticized her unrealistic fiction during it. She screamed that I was unethical for citing her novels since the debate was about objectivist psychology and had nothing to do with her fiction. She raucously threatened to walk out on the debate, and Branden had to persuade her to stay. But he also angrily alleged that I had "unethically" mentioned her novels. This was obviously ridiculous—as the nonobjectivists in the audience saw—because Rand's main presentations of objectivism *were* in *The Fountainhead, Atlas Shrugged,* and her other fiction, and her supporters mainly learned objectivist theory from her very popular novels. So I was obviously correct in criticizing their objectivist content in my debate with Branden.

Anyway, I decided to write a lengthy critique of Rand's and Branden's objectivism in a book, *Is Objectivism a Religion?*

which Lyle Stuart published in 1968 and which I thought would widely publicize the philosophy and practice of REBT and its radical differences from all the major objectivist dogmas. I thought that even many students of the Nathaniel Branden Institute would read my book and be convinced.

How wrong I was! Unfortunately, all hell broke loose between Rand and Branden while my book was about to hit the bookstores. They vituperatively broke with each other when Branden finally confessed that he had for years been sexually unfaithful to his mistress, Ayn Rand, thirty years his senior, and was practically living with a very young woman, Patrecia, with whom he had been madly in love for a couple of years.

Hearing his belated confession, Rand went almost insane, excommunicated Branden and his institute from all alliances with her and objectivism, and excoriated him for the rest of her life. She removed his name and the names of all of his supporters from the *Objectivist* newsletter mailing list and kept an enraged picture of him going forever. As many people, including objectivists, said at that time, "Hell hath no Fury like a woman scorned." Fury was putting it mildly.

Unfortunately, with the disruption of the objectivist empire, my book got lost in the shuffle. *Is Objectivism a Religion?* was one of my best books, and for many years I received lavish praise from many people who read it. But reviewers ignored it, and it quickly went out of print. Too bad—but it got buried under an avalanche of backbiting manifestos and other scurrilous remarks, especially by Rand. Meanwhile, her books continued to be best-sellers over the years.

I recently decided to bring my writings against Rand and

objectivism up to date under the title of *Ayn Rand: Her Fascistic and Fanatically Religious Philosophy*. Read it when it is published if you want the details of politico-economic philosophy of REBT and how it radically differs from the theory and practice of Ayn Rand and her holy philosophy of objectivism. Here is a brief summary of my main points in this updated revision of my book on Ayn Rand.

1. Rand's extreme view on selfishness means that unless you can specifically help yourself by any altruistic action, it is wrong and unethical to help or save others.
2. Rand believed that self-esteem is a noble goal and that you get it by being absolutely competent and outstanding. She didn't at all buy into REBT's unconditional self-acceptance.
3. She deified laissez faire, utterly free capitalism, and abhorred any combination of it with parental or state control. She thought that a thoroughly free market would automatically solve all economic problems.
4. She was completely opposed to any kind of economic planning, even though all capitalist economies have a good deal of it.
5. She inveighed against any use of physical force but refused to acknowledge the coercive power of economic force.
6. She had paranoid ideas about liberals persecuting capitalists and upholding workers at all costs.

7. She alleged that instituting Medicare would lead to a "totalitarian dictatorship" in the United States and elsewhere.

8. Rand insisted that "to deny property rights means to turn men into property owned by the state" and gives states the "right" to treat humans as chattel and awards them no "rights" whatever.

9. She held that the slightest degree of statism is wholly bad and "is a system of institutionalized violence and perpetual civil war."

10. She violently opposed pacifism and thought peace-lovers favored slave-labor camps, torture chambers, and wholesale slaughter.

11. Rand states that man absolutely should be guided by his intellect—"not a zombie guided by feelings, instincts, urges, wishes, whims." In her own life, however, and especially her love life, she was mainly guided by her strong emotions.

12. After damning the Judeo-Christian concept of sin, Rand and objectivism violently damn all noncapitalistic, unachieving, and imperfectly thinking men and women. Few creeds damn people more than objectivism. The furthest view from Rand's mind is REBT's unconditional other-acceptance.

13. Moral perfectionism is embraced by Rand when she states that you achieve it by "unbreached rationality." If your thinking is *absolutely* sound, you are then ethical. But what *makes* it absolutely sound? Unbreached objectivism!

14. Rand's extremist views of sex includes: "Man's sexual choice is the result of his fundamental conviction. Tell me what a man finds attractive and I will tell you his entire philosophy of life." Even if he falls in love only with Miss America types?

I could go on and on with dubious convictions like those I just listed. Read my book and see. Let me conclude this section, however, by my reasons for thinking that Rand's objectivism is, although she kept calling herself a hard-headed atheist, fanatically religious.

- First of all, objectivism is a faith unfounded on fact because it is absolutistic. It invents a free market or totally uncontrolled economy, in spite of its never having existed, and insists that it is the *only* economic system that can work.
- It sees *nothing* practical or good about other economic systems.
- It exaggerates and mightily invents innumerable evils of collectivism and "proves" that it is *all* bad.
- It gives no empirical reasons for deifying pure capitalism and damning every aspect of controlled capitalism and noncapitalism and it semimystically claims that they just *are* horrible states that *absolutely must* lead to utter chaos and anarchy.
- Its propagandistic novels—especially *Atlas Shrugged*—create ideal capitalists and advocates of infallible thinking and acting that are out of this world, who can do no wrong, and whose antagonists can do no right.

They are superhuman gods and their opponents are total devils.

- The religion of objectivism includes extremism and fanaticism. Rand and her followers do not merely believe that their dogmas are valid, but they overzealously are *certain* that they are entirely superior to everyone else's politico-economic theories. In Eric Hoffer's terms, they are *true believers*.

- Rand and other dyed-in-the-wool objectivists often resort to tautological, definitional thinking. They *define* pure capitalism and utter political freedom as "good" and "true" and allege that any deviation from those "perfect" systems is "bad" and "false."

- Randian objectivists are not theological in the usual sense but are secular religionists who have holy and sacred missions, follow a sacrosanct bible (*Atlas Shrugged*) and other objectivist rituals, and feel thoroughly ashamed of themselves when they fail to consistently follow the "right path." Branden, for example, beat himself mercilessly when he was sexually unfaithful to Ayn Rand and failed to follow the "right" objectivist behavior. When he broke with her, many objectivists berated themselves for having falsely followed Branden's teachings.

- Like most religionists, Rand, Branden, and their followers thoroughly follow the sacrament of self-esteem or conditioned self-acceptance. They define their principles as infinitely superior to other philosophers and see themselves as noble, "superior" persons for achieving this delectable summit. Then they are beyond reproach, can do no wrong, and will reach the objectivist heaven without having to die to get there. Their self-deification is tautologically assured.

As you can see from this summary, Ayn Rand and her objectivist philosophy have largely opposing views to the theory and practice of REBT. This doesn't mean that either of us is right and the other wrong, but it does show that REBT has a distinct politico-economic set of attitudes. In contrast to Randism—and to a number of other world views—it holds that its therapeutic aspects include a set of teachings that effectively help people feel better, get better, and stay better. In contrast, I would (prejudicedly) say that Ayn Rand's personal and philosophic model was deeply thought out and forcefully promulgated. In many ways, it was original, brilliant, and convincing. It still turns on thousands of readers every year. But in the REBT view, it tends to encourage them to be mentally and emotionally less healthy than they were before starting to follow it. This means, in my opinion, that Randians, in adopting objectivism, add to the fanaticism, bigotry, and emotional disturbance to which they already are addicted.

Which raises another important point. I wrote a widely cited essay on intellectual fascism in the original version of *Sex without Guilt* in 1958 and included it again in *Sex without Guilt in the Twentieth Century* in 2003. Its main thesis is that we think of fascism as a political and economic policy—as shown in Mussolini's Italian state and

Hitler's German Third Reich. Actually, it has been widespread in "liberal" regions, such as America, for more than fifty years in the form of intellectual fascism.

What is intellectual fascism? I describe it in *Sex without Guilt* and in appendix A in this book. Very briefly, it is a philosophy that denigrates and punishes people when they do not live up to the "good" and "noble" intellectual standards of their educated and cultured detractors. Thus, intellectual fascists in the United States (and much of Western civilization) scorn "philistines" who are ignorant, stupid, blue-collared, and less sophisticated than they are.

Ayn Rand and her staunch objectivist supporters are typical intellectual fascists. They, and they alone, have the "right" social, political, and economic attitudes and practices; those who in any way fall below these high standards are rightly to be despised and boycotted. As Rand frequently refers to them, they are "thugs," "vermin," "worms," "loafers," "bums," and other lower-than-low individuals. For sure! They deserve, of course, to be fought and boycotted but also obliterated from the human race.

Now we could ask the question: Were devout Randians born and reared to be seriously disturbed people who *therefore* adopted rabid objectivist attitudes? Or did their rigid allegiance to objectivism *make* them emotionally disturbed?

I would say both/and rather than either/or. A large number of fervent objectivists I personally encountered (not merely as clients but as acquaintances) I diagnosed as having severe personality disorders all their lives. But some converts to objectivism I saw as "nice neurotics" who *became* seriously bigoted and disordered *after* their conversion to Randianism. They *adopted* profound intellectual (and other) fascism when they converted to objectivism.

What about Ayn Rand herself? Though I never actually met her—because she avoided Roger Callahan's and Lee Shulman's urgent invitations to meet with me—I had enough secondhand knowledge of her to see her as severely personality disordered from adolescence onward. But I also (prejudicedly) saw that her fanatical involvement with objectivism helped her be more disturbed than she otherwise would have been. Also her obsessive-compulsive affair with Nathaniel Branden didn't help make her saner!

To sum up: Branden at first viewed objectivism and REBT as quite similar theories and practices, but that seems to have been wishful thinking. In many ways, as I have shown in this chapter and as other observers have indicated, the two systems have little in common and are at odds in almost all important ways. Let us hope so!

11

A Consideration of "Rational" and "Irrational" Spirituality

When psychotherapy began to be popular in the first part of the twentieth century, it did not often recommend that people help themselves with religion and spirituality. Quite the contrary! Carl Jung was unusual in his favoring of mystical attitudes and techniques, but Sigmund Freud and Alfred Adler were in opposite camps, as were emotionally oriented therapists like Wilhelm Reich and Fritz Perls and, of course, behaviorists like John B. Watson and Fred Skinner. A survey of the religious and spiritual beliefs of the members of the American Academy of Psychotherapists in the 1960s showed that more than 80 percent of them were not religious and disfavored spiritual activities in therapy.

Later in the 1900s, psychotherapists and counselors considerably changed, and several books and scores of professional articles began to take favorable and even enthusiastic spiritual leanings. This was because some studies found that although it could hardly be proven that gods, spirits, or supernatural entities existed, some distinct evidence showed that therapy clients and other people with emotional problems improved their mental health and physical functioning when they definitely *believed* in the power of religious and spiritual faith. Whatever spiritual convictions they had—and some of them indeed seemed to be far-fetched from a scientific point of view—their religious and mystical faith worked.

As I indicated in my chapter of this book on religion, this was predictable on the basis of REBT theory—which says that it's not just harsh "reality" that bothers people but their *view* of it. If, then, they have a pronounced *view* of spiritual forces helping them, they frequently will follow this attitude and thereby often "get" help from these (quite possibly) nonexistent forces. Strange—but empirically verifiable.

At any rate, seeing this evidence, all sorts of writers jumped on the bandwagon to endorse "spiritual therapy." Not only, as you would expect, the regular devotees of spiritualism, who now endorsed it more than ever but also empiricists (including agnostics and atheists) were on a seeming similar jaunt. Thus, Carl Sagan and Richard Dawkins said that they were still staunch empirical scientists but that the natural observable order—such as the stars and human inventiveness and creative thinking—could justifiably be viewed enthusiastically with respect, awe, and honor. Sagan wrote:

> This view showed that natural events could be seen to have a "spiritual" or emotional quality. Your firmly believing that supernatural mystical forces were "real," when they probably never existed, could nicely affect you in a similar way to your holding that faith in (a dubiously existing) God or shaman could benefit you. Marvelous!

The question therefore arises: Had we better not clearly differentiate between old-time "spiritual beliefs" in gods and other magic forces and modern definitions of "spirituality" that seem to consist of meaningful experiences that have no supernaturalism connected with them?

Take conventional, old-time spiritualism first. People who have these kinds of convictions have no empirical evidence to present, but they still have faith in the helpfulness of priests, ministers, rabbis, prayer, personal intuition, rituals, their own grandiosity, and so forth. Empirically, this kind of magical faith unfounded on fact cannot be validated and is quite probably illusory. The fact that it *may* work out in practice is true, but the fact that it most often doesn't work is also true. For the one person who conquers cancer because she prays to Mary Baker Eddy and the Christian Science scriptures, how many die sooner because they fail to get proper medical care? Quite a few, you can be reasonably sure!

There's the rub. Hard-headed facts show that some people benefit from having unfactual faith in supernatural cures when, in all probability, the gods and magical helpers to whom they devoutly pray do not actually exist. But what about the faith-inspired *harm* that many true believers promote? By what kind of studies are we to measure *that*? How are we to evaluate the religious and spiritual faith of the Christian Scientists who have cancer and who pray to Mary Baker Eddy and her church in vain? Questioning these dead people isn't too practical!

My arguments, however, do not contradict the virtues of the "spiritual" techniques that include no supernatural elements and have been endorsed by an increasing number of purposive philosophies and actions that have been recommended, especially during the last decade. If you have these "spiritual" attitudes, you may endorse the following behaviors:

1. Make an effort to lead a well-balanced rather than a one-sided life.
2. When you are behaving in a disturbed manner, acknowledge this and try to improve.
3. Accept your disturbances, and don't blame yourself for having them.
4. Have a present- and future-oriented attitude instead of allowing yourself to be preoccupied with your past.
5. Be a responsible person who cultivates good character.
6. Do your best to have a good sense of humor.
7. Work at increasing your self-discipline.
8. Be active and energetic.
9. Have considerable courage in the face of difficulties.
10. Follow your own bliss in spite of the criticism of others who want you to follow theirs.
11. Choose reason rather than immediate short-term gratification.
12. Be optimistic and hopeful.
13. Have compassion and love for others.
14. Achieve intimacy with some other people.
15. Be creative and preferably original.
16. Have integrity and honesty.

In the field of psychotherapy, therapists have especially recommended these "spiritual" values:

1. Try to improve yourself but also subscribe to some special, unusual, or higher than selfish meaning.
2. Try to achieve an unusual or higher state of consciousness or awareness.
3. Achieve a higher degree of intellectual power.
4. Acquire an outstanding useful meaning or purpose in life.
5. Acquire unconditional acceptance, love, and forgiveness for yourself.
6. Have unusual social interests, empathy, and compassion for others.
7. Dislike and try to change the world's difficulties and misfortunes, but thoroughly accept those that you cannot change.
8. Be profoundly optimistic and have considerable hope for the future.
9. Try to live up to your potential but not evaluate your worth by your achievements.
10. Have a strong belief in your self-healing and self-helping abilities.
11. Have a vital, absorbing interest in some area and work hard to implement that interest.

In reviewing the recent literature, I came across these recommended "spiritual" goals and a few more. As you will note, most of them are similar to the goals of REBT and other modern modes of psychotherapy. I personally endorse almost all of them, and I favor them in my individual and group therapy sessions with my clients.

The question remains: Does it make much sense to call these therapeutic goals "spiritual?" I doubt it. Although they are profoundly *meaningful* and *purposive* aims, they are becoming more common than ever today and have few of the *unique* or *special* aspects that the word *spiritual* implies. In the old meaning of the term, everyday humans are not going to be very spiritual until and if they ascend to heaven. But some of us—including me—do not exactly believe in heaven, and, in a sense, those who preach the old-time spiritualism really do. Aren't the devotees of old-time "spiritual" behavior in some ways significantly different from the espousers of modern "spiritualistic" advocates?

I think that the two groups are far from alike. The old-time "spiritual" advocates may be called transcendentalists because they transcend, or go beyond, natural living processes. By nature, as well as by social learning, we are limited and restricted people—common humans. Therefore, we see only the empirical facts that our senses observe: material things and other living creatures. We observe them with our eyes, ears, nose, mouth, and kinesthetic attributes—not with *special* senses beyond that. In other words, we are distinctly material, and if we have a nonmaterial essence or soul, we cannot observe it. We can infer it, imagine it, but not empirically get in touch with it.

This means that if we are really spiritual in the conventional sense, we have a *special*, nonsensory way of reaching our soul. Our special way *transcends* our regular sensory ways so that "spiritual" means "transcendental." Although we may be transcendental and not exactly religious—for we may not believe in any God—transcendental still seems to mean faith in some kind of power that is beyond human power—such as faith in prayer, faith in our own unusual power, faith in the universe, or faith in some other nonobservable things. Transcendental knowledge is *higher* than ordinary knowledge. It includes a *higher* form of consciousness. It may include asceticism and giving up of desire and a state of no-mind or of no meaning. It is hard to describe what it really means because regular meaning is seen with our mind and transcendental goes beyond mind and meaning—to what? That's very hard to say. Mind and intellect are presumably a function of the brain, and transcendental, intuitive people presumably transcend their bodies, brains, intellect, and who knows what else. It is hard to imagine what is left!

Religionists believe that there *is* a God or Higher Power who loves and will take care of them. Transcendentalists may not go along with that idea but seem to believe that they *have* higher powers to perceive what the rest of us can't and thereby *become* higher than other ordinary humans. I definitely don't believe any God or other superhumans exist; I don't believe that I am God or any special superhuman entity. Either of those beliefs could easily lead to disillusionment and depression. Stubbornly refusing to give them up leads to Pollyannaism. Who needs either or these two afflictions?

Although the meaning of "spirituality" has been revised in recent years so that it is becoming almost synonymous with practical therapeutic teachings, this is far from true in the cases of therapists and writers who still follow old-time "spiritual" directives. Their recommendations always were and still are, I might humorously say, out of this world. They basically evoke supernatural and empirically unconfirmable principles and practices. They encourage behaviors that may lead to some benefits for devout believers but also may directly or subtly harm emotionally disturbed and other people. For example:

1. Conventional "spiritual" beliefs, because they are empirically unconfirmable or confirmable, are absolutistic and rigid. Absolutism and rigidity, as REBT keeps showing, often lead to unrealism and to impaired mental and emotional health.
2. To seek and work for "higher" nonmaterial and less selfish causes is purposive and enjoyable—as long as you are not obsessively-compulsively convinced that they make you a special person who is essentially better than other unspecial people. You then have *conditional* self-acceptance that may cover up serious feelings of worthlessness.
3. Work for the laudable value of social interest or REBT's unconditional other-acceptance may be taken to extremes and done to prove that you are a *special* person who will go to heaven after your stint on earth is done. Good deeds do *not* make you a noble person.

4. Having an outstanding goal or purpose in life has great advantages and has been recommended by REBT and existential therapy for many years. But it doesn't ennoble you and can again become obsessive-compulsive. Many people get by happily with no vital absorbing goal. You can *desire* to have one and choose it, but you don't have to make it a *dire necessity* that will boost your ego.

5. Achieving "spirituality" by having a profound belief that all things, animate and inanimate, are unified and are integrally integrated is partly true—because as a human you cannot exist without other living creatures and without an external environment. But if you believe that you are wholly at one with all living and nonliving parts of the universe—as some spiritual followers of Lao-Tsu do—you will be unrealistic, will refuse to use animals and objects for healthy living, and will hardly survive.

6. Striving for a state of higher or pure consciousness may help you expand your mind and widen your feelings. But *pure* consciousness probably is unachievable. It would be divorced from your body, brain, and sensory-nervous system and akin to a disembodied soul. You can imagine having it but never have it. If you had pure consciousness, what would it be conscious *of?* Itself? It would truly be unique. But how would it make you a spiritual, Godlike *person?*

7. Giving up all sensory and other pleasure for a complete ascetic life may reduce your desires and worries. But

what kind of spirituality is that? You wouldn't even *know* that you had achieved spirituality.

8. As I have noted, giving up your dire need for pleasure, success, and the approval of others may have real advantages in reducing your anxiety, depression, anger, and low frustration tolerance when you fail to get what you think you *absolutely need*. But bringing about a state of desirelessness—which in spiritual language is called nirvana—is probably impossible, would result in your demise, and might well be a great bore. Instead of enlightenment, it sounds pretty dull! If accomplished for any length of time, you might feel no pain or misery, but it would end your personal life as well as your social relationships. Some "spirituality!"

As can be seen if you consider the above disadvantages of conventional spirituality, goals and values that go far beyond human purposes, that cannot be empirically seen and evaluated, and that include supernatural factors may have certain advantages. If you think they will benefit you, by all means try to achieve them. But although you may strongly believe that these kinds of spiritual achievements will lead you to unalloyed enlightenment and joy, this is questionable. Try out these extreme spiritual goals and see for yourself.

If, as a therapist or a helping friend, you work with extreme believers in spirituality, you are probably not going to persuade them to moderate their spiritual views, and you can let them hold on to them. I am a distinctly secular humanist who doesn't believe in anything supernatural, transcendental, or higher-than-human. But I have worked with many substance abusers who are absolutely certain that a Higher Power exists and cares for them. Although I think they are deluded in this respect, I let them keep this conventional spiritual view and use the other aspects of REBT to help them. This normally works quite well.

I also use modern, revised "spirituality" with these and other clients. Doing so, I encourage them to strongly have profoundly meaningful, purposive, spirited, and long-range goals, such as those I listed earlier. These could also be called REBT goals or aims of "rational spirituality."

As an example, I worked with a thirty-nine-year-old man who had been compulsively drinking to sedate his anxiety and his shyness about dating women since the age of fifteen. Ronald had sporadically attended Alcoholics Anonymous meetings several times but always went back to drinking when he was shy and withdrawn at office parties and other gatherings where there were attractive women. He definitely believed in AA's "Higher Power" but berated himself considerably for inconsistently heeding God's injunctions to stop drinking. His "Higher Power" was indeed powerful, but he was so weak that he kept ignoring its sensible encouragement to stop drinking. Even with God's help, he was helpless and was stubbornly refusing to follow his deity.

I didn't contradict Ronald's belief in the goodness of God and his own badness for stubbornly resisting the Higher Power's help, though I was sorely tempted at times to show him that the God he believed in was a very weak deity whose "power" was questionable. I felt that Ronald had better stop relying on any supernatural help and therefore take his *own* power into his hands and use it to stop drinking. But I thought that Ronald wouldn't accept my interpretation, so I shut my big mouth.

Instead, I used several main REBT methods with him, particularly unconditional self-acceptance. I showed him that any helpful "Higher Power" would thoroughly accept him even if he never gave up drinking and that with a caring God and with his own USA—which he could consider as a fine gift from God—he was always able to accept himself. USA was a marvelous potentiality of *all* people, including himself. Ronald finally saw this, and, as REBT postulates, he was able to see that his drinking was stupid and destructive but that *he* was not worthless for indulging in it. We also, he and I, helped him see that his shyness and weakness about approaching women stemmed from his overwhelming *need* to succeed with them and that when he still *desired* to succeed but didn't *have to* do so, much of his shyness vanished.

At the same time, I used REBT's revised mode of spirituality with Ronald. I helped him have a vital absorbing purpose in life—not only to stop drinking but also to have the goal of being unanxious about his shyness and about his falling back to the drinking. I helped him devote himself to AA to help himself and to have the "higher" goal of helping other alcoholics. Although AA wouldn't make him a sponsor of others because of his bad track record, he unofficially began to help several people with their own weak indulgences. I also encouraged Ronald to give up his pessimism about stopping drinking and to take a more optimistic view of his ability to stop and stay stopped.

In several ways, then, I recommended that Ronald be spiritual in his goals and purposes and thereby to become stronger in his fight against social anxiety and his determination to increase his antidrinking thoughts, feelings, and actions. At the end of our fourteen months of REBT, he reported that he was delighted to maintain his sobriety but even more delighted to be in control of himself and his various weaknesses. He especially liked his minimal self-deprecation.

To sum up, REBT and my use of it can accept the conventional, God-implied spirituality of millions of people who find this chosen element of their lives distinctly helpful. But it also encourages a nonsuperhuman view of striving that features profoundly purposive, meaningful, enthusiastic, and spirited spirituality, which we may call "rational spirituality."

12

Conclusion

I have attempted to show in this book the philosophical, religious, social, political, and economic aspects of Rational Emotive Behavior Therapy. All psychotherapies have core philosophies behind their espousal of some of their techniques and their neglect of other techniques. REBT, in particular, was inspired by philosophy and has openly stayed with its inspiration.

It consequently has pronounced theories of how people are born and raised with strong tendencies to disturb themselves; how they use their cognitive, emotional, and behavioral predispositions to do so; and what they can specifically do to suffer less and lead a happier existence. REBT's philosophy of psychotherapy consciously incorporates a philosophy of living. It assumes that if people's basic values and attitudes encourage them to be mentally and emotionally healthy, they will still suffer from many frustrations and misfortunes. But they will not be, as they frequently are today, overwhelmed by anxiety, depression, and rage about these adversities. They will be much better able to face the adversities they often encounter, to reduce them appreciably, and to cope with those that still remain.

As a human, you are a constructivist in that you partly choose your desires and avoidances, you can observe and assess whether or not they work out well, and you can change or retain your choices. Not easily or completely, of course, for you are restricted by your biological limitations and by the strong influences of your social learning. Still, if you use your unique ability to think about your thinking, about your feelings, and about your doings, you can strongly (emotionally) and persistently (actively) change and improve them.

The theory of Rational Emotive Behavior Therapy holds that you can use your ability to choose—which is often called your free will—when you particularly see that thinking, feeling, and behaving are integrally connected. When you think, you also feel and act. When you feel, you also think and act. When you act, you also think and feel. Three in one!

Therefore, if you want to change your dysfunctional ways, you first think—decide—to modify them. But you had better determine, strongly and emotionally, to do so, and you had better do so actively and behaviorally—push, push, push to change. You *powerfully and forcefully* act on what you decide is your best interest.

Aside from disturbance, if you want to change a good part of your life—say, eat *healthier* food—you had better think *strongly* and *determinedly* about doing so, to keep *pushing* yourself to change. REBT encourages you to think *and* feel *and* act to modify your poor choices—but also to think, feel, and act on the good aspects of your life that you want to improve.

Again, you can use REBT *in general* and not merely *therapeutically*. How? By your working in social, political, economic, and other ways to gain and keep unconditional self-acceptance, unconditional other-acceptance, and unconditional life-acceptance. Reread chapter 2 and chapters 9 and 10 to see how to do this.

I specifically emphasize the "road to tolerance" in this book, for it is easy for you, like most people, to think, feel, and act intolerantly—to choose your desires, goals, and values and hold them rigidly, one-sidedly, bigotedly, absolutistically, and fanatically. Why? Because you were partly born and partly reared to go to extremes and to think in all-or-nothing, overgeneralized terms. Your intolerance and your extremism often make you disturbed; your disturbance solidifies your intolerance. Reciprocally!

REBT, like some other therapies, is largely a form of tolerance training. It encourages you to think, feel, and act the ways you want—but warns against rigidity and fanaticism. Reread chapters 2, 9, 10, and 11 to see why. Actually, the road to tolerance consists of a number of roads, three of which are very important in REBT and in your life:

- *Unconditional self-acceptance* means that you do not tolerate your destructive demands—your *absolutistic shoulds, oughts, and musts*—but replace them with *flexible preferences*: "I would distinctly *like* to do well and win the approval of others, but I don't *have to* do so. If and when

I fail and get rejected, I can always accept *myself*, my *being*, while remaining intolerant of some of my *behaviors*.

- *Unconditional other-acceptance* means that you do not tolerate the antisocial and sabotaging actions of other people, and you try to help them change. But you always accept *them*, their personhood, and you never damn their total *selves*. You tolerate their *humanity* while disagreeing with some of their *actions*.

- *Unconditional life-acceptance* means that you deplore adversities and injustices and do your best to rectify them. But when you can't change inevitable misfortunes, you un-upsetably accept them and do not enrage, panic, or depress yourself about them.

While trying your best to tolerate and stop damning your flawed self, other people's personhood, and life's inevitable troubles, you strongly remain determined to encourage and to work for your own and other's improvement and for the world's peaceful development. Is this kind of tolerance worth your—and my!—thought, feeling, and behaving? I truly hope so!

Appendix A
Intellectual Fascism

If *fascism* is defined as the arbitrary belief that individuals possessing certain traits (such as those who are white, Aryan, or male) are intrinsically superior to individuals possessing certain other traits (such as those who are black, Jewish, or female), and that therefore the "superior" individuals should have distinct politico-social privileges, then the vast majority of American liberals and so-called antifascists are actually intellectual fascists. In fact, the more politico-economically liberal our citizens are, the more intellectually fascistic they often tend to be.

Intellectual fascism—in accordance with the above definition—is the arbitrary belief that individuals possessing certain traits (such as those who are intelligent, cultured, artistic, creative, or achieving) are intrinsically superior to individuals possessing certain other traits (such as those who are uneducated, uncultured, unartistic, uncreative, or unachieving). The reason why the belief of the intellectual fascist, like that of the politico-social fascist, is arbitrary is simple: there is no objective evidence to support it. At bottom, it is based on value judgments or prejudices that are definitional in character and are not empirically validatable, nor is it falsifiable. It is a value chosen by a group of prejudiced people—and not necessarily by a majority.

This is not to deny that verifiable differences exist among various individuals. They certainly do. Women, in some ways, are different from men; short people do differ from tall ones; stupid individuals can be separated from bright ones. Anyone who denies this, whatever his or her good intentions, is simply not accepting reality.

Human differences, moreover, usually have their distinct advantages and disadvantages. Under tropical conditions, the darkly pigmented blacks seem to fare better than do the lightly pigmented whites. At the same time, many blacks and fewer whites become afflicted with sickle cell anemia. When it comes to playing basketball, tall men are generally superior to short ones. But as jockeys and coxswains, the undersized have their day. For designing and operating electric computers, a plethora of gray matter is a vital necessity; for driving a car for long distances, it is likely to prove a real handicap.

Let us face the fact, then, that under certain conditions some human traits are more advantageous—or "better"—than some other traits. Whether we approve the fact or not, they are. All people in today's world may be created free, but they certainly are not created equal.

Granting that this is so, the important question is, does the possession of a specific advantageous endowment make an individual a better human? Or more concretely, does the fact that someone is an excellent athlete, artist, author, or achiever make him or her a better person? Consciously or unconsciously, both the politico-social and the intellectual fascist say yes to these questions.

This is gruesomely clear when we consider politico-social or lower-order fascists, for they honestly and openly not only tell themselves and the world that being white, Aryan, male, or a member of the state-supported party, is a grand and glorious thing, but, simultaneously, they just as honestly and openly admit that they despise, loathe, and consider as scum of the earth individuals who are not so fortunate as to be in these select categories. Lower-order fascists at least have the conscious courage of their own convictions.

Not so, alas, intellectual or higher-order fascists, for they almost invariably pride themselves on their liberality, humanitarianism, and lack of arbitrary prejudice against certain classes of people. But underneath, just because they have no insight into their fascistic beliefs, they are often more vicious, in their social effects, than their lower-order counterparts.

Take, by way of illustration, two well-educated, presumably liberal, intelligent people in our culture who are arguing with each other about some point. What, out of irritation and disgust, is one likely to call the other? A "filthy black," a "dirty Jew bastard," or a "black-eyed runt"? Heavens, no. But a "stupid idiot," a "nincompoop," or a "misinformed numbskull"? By all means, yes. And will the note of venom of utter despisement that is in the detractor's voice be any different from that in the voice of the out-and-out fascist with his racial, religious, and political epithets? Honestly, now: will it?

Suppose that the individual against whom a well-educated, presumably liberal, intelligent person aims scorn actually is stupid or misinformed. Is this a crime? Should she, perforce, curl up and die because she is so afflicted? Is she an utterly worthless, valueless blackguard for not possessing the degree of intelligence and knowledge that her detractor thinks she should possess? And yet—let us be ruthlessly honest with ourselves, now—isn't this exactly what the presumably liberal person is saying and implying: that the individual whose traits she dislikes doesn't deserve to live? Isn't this what we (for it is not hard to recognize our own image here, is it?) frequently allege when we argue with, criticize, and judge others in our everyday living?

The facts, in regard to higher-order fascism, are just as clear as those in regard to lower-order prejudice. For just as everyone in our society cannot be, except through the process of arbitrary genocide or "eugenic" elimination, Aryan, tall, or white, so cannot everyone be bright, artistically talented, or successful in some profession. In fact, even if we deliberately bred only highly intelligent and artistically endowed individuals to each other and forced the rest of the human race to die off, we still would be far from obtaining a race of universal achievers, since, by definition, topflight achievement can only be attained by a relatively few leaders in most fields of endeavor and is a relative rather than an absolute possibility.

The implicit goals of intellectual fascism, then, are, at least in today's world, impractical and utopian. Everyone cannot be endowed with artistic or intellectual genius; only a small minority can be. And if we demand that all be in that minority, to what are we automatically condemning those who clearly cannot be? Obviously: to being blamed and despised for their "deficiencies," to being lower-class citizens, to having self-hatred and minimal self-acceptance.

Even this, however, hardly plumbs the inherent viciousness of intellectual fascism. For whereas lower-order or politico-economic fascism at least serves as a form of neurotic defensiveness for those who uphold its tenets, higher-order fascism fails to provide such defenses and actually destroys them. Thus, politico-social fascists believe that others are to be despised for not having certain "desirable" traits but that they themselves are to be applauded for having them. From a psychological standpoint, they compensate for their own underlying feelings of inadequacy by insisting that they are superadequate and that those who are not like them are subhumans.

Intellectual fascists start out with a similar assumption but more often than not get blown to bits by their own homemade explosives. For although they can at first assume that they are bright, talented, and potentially achieving, they must eventually prove that they are. Because, in the last analysis, they tend to define *talent* and *intelligence* in terms of concrete achievement, and because outstanding achievement in our society is mathematically restricted to a few, they rarely can have real confidence in their own possession of the values they have arbitrarily deified.

To make matters still worse, intellectual fascists frequently demand of themselves, as well as others, perfect competence and universal achievement. If they are excellent mathematicians or dancers, they demand that they be the most accomplished. If they are outstanding scientists or manufacturers, they also must be first-rate painters or writers. If they are fine poets, they not only need to be the finest but likewise must be great lovers, drawing room wits, and political experts. Naturally, only being human, they fail at many or most of these ventures. And then—O, poetic justice!—they apply to themselves the same excoriations and despisements that they apply to others when they fail to be universal geniuses.

However righteous their denials, therefore—and even though those readers who by now are not squirming with guilt are probably screaming with indignation, I will determinedly continue—the typical politico-social "liberals" of our day are fascistic in several significant ways. They arbitrarily define certain human traits as "good" or "superior"; they automatically exclude most others from any possibility of achieving their "good" standards; they scorn, combat, and in many ways persecute those who do not live up to these capricious goals; and, finally, in most instances they more or less fail to live up to their own definitional standards and bring down neurotic self-pity and blame on their own heads.

Let me give a case in point that I deliberately take not from my psychotherapeutic practice (since, as one might expect, it is replete with cases of all kinds of self-haters) but from my presumably less neurotic acquaintanceship. It is the case of a man I have known for many years who, partly because of his long-standing union connections and the fact that his parents were killed by the Nazis, prides himself on his antifascist views. This individual, however, not only tries to avoid associating with people whom he considers unintelligent (which, of course, is his privilege, just as it is the privilege of a musician to try to associate mainly with other musicians) but also goes into long diatribes against almost everybody he meets because they are "so terribly stupid" or "real idiots" or "utterly impossible." He gets quite upset whenever he encounters people who turn out to be below his accepted standards of intelligence, and he says that he cannot understand "why they let people like that live. Surely the world would be much better off without such dopes."

This same individual, as I would have predicted from seeing many clients with similar views, has for many years been completely ineffective in his own desire to write short stories. Every time he reads over a few paragraphs he has written, he finds them to be "stupid," "inconsequential," or "trite," and he stops right there. He obviously is trying to write not because he enjoys doing so or feels that he'd like to express himself, but mainly because he has to be admired, accepted, and thought intelligent by other people, particularly by other writers. His intellectual fascism not only prejudices all his human relationships but also sabotages his own creativity and potential happiness. His name, I contend, is legion.

What is the alternative? Assuming that intellectual fascism exists on a wide scale today, and that it does enormous harm and little good to people's relations with themselves and others, what philosophy of living are they to set up in its place? Surely, you may well ask, I am not suggesting an uncritical, sentimental equalitarianism, whereunder everyone would fully accept and hobnob with everyone else and where no one would attempt to excel or perfect himself at anything. No, I am not.

I feel, on the contrary, that significant human differences (as well as samenesses) exist; that they add much variety and zest to living, and that one human may sensibly cultivate the company of another just because this other is different from, and perhaps in certain specific respects superior to, others. I feel, at the same time, that one's worth as a human being is not to be measured in terms of one's popularity, success, achievement, intelligence, or any other such trait but solely in terms of one's humanity.

More positively stated: I espouse the seemingly revolutionary doctrine, which actually goes back many hundreds of years and is partially incorporated into the philosophies of Jesus of Nazareth and several other religious leaders, that people are worthwhile merely because they exist, not because they exist in an intelligent, cultured, artistic, achieving, or other way. If any particular person decides to pursue a certain goal, such as excelling at basketball or astrophysics, then it may be better for this purpose that he or she be tall, intelligent, supple, or something else. But if the main purpose of humans is, as I think it can be, living in some kind of satisfactory way, then it is highly desirable that they live and enjoy simply by acting, doing, and being and not by acting, doing, or being outstanding.

Let us get this matter perfectly straight, since it is the easiest thing to muddle and confuse. I am not in any manner, shape, or form opposed to people's trying to achieve a given goal and to this end consistently practicing some task and trying to keep bettering their performances. I believe, in fact, that most men and women cannot live too happily without some kind of goal, direction, or vital interest in solving problems or completing long-range projects.

I still maintain, however, that the fact that people achieve, produce, solve, or complete projects is not to be used as a measure of their intrinsic value. They may be happier, healthier, richer, or more confident if they successfully paint, write, or manufacture a useful product. But they will not be, nor is it desirable that they see themselves as, better *people*.

In Rational Emotive Behavior Therapy (REBT), we encourage you to refrain from rating your *self*, your *totality*, your *essence*, or your *being* at all—but instead to rate *only* your acts, deeds, and performances.

Why had you better not rate your *self* or your *essence*? For several reasons:

1. Rating your *self* or your *you*-ness is an overgeneralization and is virtually impossible to do accurately. You *are* (consist of) literally millions of acts, deeds, and traits during your lifetime. Even if you were fully aware of all these performances and characteristics (which you never will be) and were able to give each of them a rating (say, from zero to one hundred), *how* would you rate each one, for what *purpose*, and under what *conditions*? Even if you could accurately rate *all* your millions of acts, how could you get a *mean* or *global* rating of the *you* who performs them? Not very easily!

2. Just as your deeds and characteristics constantly change (today you play tennis or chess or the stock market very well and tomorrow quite badly), so does your *self* change. Even if you could, at any one second, somehow give your *totality* a legitimate rating, this rating would keep changing constantly as you did new things and had more experiences. Only after your death could you give your *self* a final and stable rating. Perhaps!

3. What is the *purpose* of rating your *self* or achieving *ego* aggrandizement or *self*-esteem? Obviously, to make you feel better than other people: to grandiosely deify yourself, to be holier than thou, and to rise to heaven in a golden chariot. Nice work—if you can do it! But since self-esteem seems to be highly correlated with what Albert Bandura calls self-efficacy, you can only have stable ego-strength when (a) you do well, (b) you know you will continue to do well, and (c) you have a guarantee that you will always equal or best others in important performances in the present and future. Well, unless you are truly perfect, lots of luck on *those* aspirations!

4. Although rating your performances and comparing them to those of others has real value—because it will help you improve your efficacy and presumably increase your happiness—rating your *self* and insisting that you must be a good and adequate *person* will (unless you, again, are perfect!) almost inevitably

result in your being anxious when you do any important thing badly, depressed when you do behave poorly, hostile when others outperform you, and self-pitying when conditions interfere with your doing as well as you think you *should*. In addition to these neurotic and debilitating feelings, you will almost certainly suffer from serious behavioral problems, such as procrastination, withdrawal, shyness, phobias, obsessions, inertia, and inefficiency.

For these reasons, as well as others I have outlined elsewhere, rating or measuring your *self* or your *ego* will tend to make you anxious, miserable, and ineffective. By all means, rate your *acts* and try (undesperately!) to do well. For you may be happier, healthier, richer, or more achievement-confident (confident that you *can* achieve) if you perform adequately. But you will not be, nor had you better define yourself as, a better *person*.

If you insist on rating your *self* or your *personhood* at all—which REBT advises you *not* to do—you had better conceive of yourself as being valuable or worthwhile just because you are human, because you are alive, because you exist. Preferably, don't rate your *self* or your *being* at *all*, and then you won't get into any philosophic or scientific difficulties. But if you do use inaccurate, overgeneralized self-ratings, such as "I am a good person," "I am worthwhile," or "I like myself," say "I am a good person because I exist and not because I do something special." Then you will not be rating yourself in a rigid, bigoted, authoritarian—that is, fascistic—manner.

Human traits are good for a purpose, and are not, in, of, by, and for themselves, good or bad, virtuous or evil. Intelligence is good for problem solving, aesthetic sensitivity for enjoyment, persistence for achievement, honesty for putting others at their ease, courage for facing dangers with equanimity. But intelligence, aesthetic sensitivity, persistence, honesty, courage, or any other purposeful trait is not, except by arbitrary definition, an end in itself nor an absolute good. And as soon as such a trait is defined as a good thing in itself, all nonpossessors of that trait tend to be labeled as evil or worthless. Such an arbitrary, overgeneralized labeling, again, is fascistic.

What, then, can be taken as a valid measure of a person's worth? If being intelligent or artistic or honest or what you will does not render him or her "good" or "worthwhile," what does?

Nothing, actually. All human "worth" or "value" is simply a *choice*, a *decision*. We *choose* to rate our *selves* or to not do so. Almost always (because that seems to be our nature or innate predisposition) we *decide* to give ourselves global ratings. And we *select* standards to use for this rating. Thus, we *choose* to rate ourselves as "good people" because (1) we perform well; (2) we have good, moral character traits; (3) we win the approval of others; (4) we are members of a favored group, community, or nation; or (5) we believe in some deity (e.g., Jehovah, Jesus, or Allah), whom we are convinced created us and rates us globally for our "good" or "bad" accomplishments. We assume that God, too, is fascistic!

All these "criteria" of our "worth," "value," or "goodness" are actually arbitrary and are valid because we *choose* to believe them so. None of them, except by our *belief* in them, is empirically confirmable or falsifiable. Some work well and some badly—that is, bring us more or less happiness and greater or lesser disturbance. If we are wise, therefore, we will select those criteria of our "worth" or "value" that bring us the best results.

According to REBT, the best or most effective criterion of our human worth would probably be *no* self rating—yes, *no* measure of our *self* or our *ego*. For then we would *only* rate our behaviors and traits and thereby strive for continued aliveness and enjoyment—and not for deification or devilification. And because self-ratings are overgeneralizations that are impossible to validate, we would be philosophically sounder—and nonfascistic.

If you do, however, choose to rate your *self* or your *totality*, why not rate it in terms of your *aliveness* and your *enjoyment*? Try, for example, this philosophy: "I am alive and I choose to stay alive and to try to enjoy my existence. I will rate my *aliveness*, my *existence* as 'good' because that is my choice, and if my aliveness truly becomes too painful or unenjoyable, I may rationally *choose* to end it. Meanwhile, I value my existence (my *be*-ing) simply because I am alive and, while so alive, I can sense, feel, think, and act. This I select as my 'real' worth: my humanity, my aliveness, my present cheating of nonexistence."

From choosing to value your aliveness, your existence, you can also choose various subvalues. You can decide, for example, to be happily, vitally, maximally, or fully alive. You can judge that if it is good for you to be alive and happy, it is also good if you help others enjoy their existence (and to enjoy yours with them). You can plan to live healthfully, peacefully, and productively. Once you *choose* to see living as "worthwhile," you will probably also choose to live in a social group, to be intimate with some others, to work productively, and to engage in several recreational pursuits. These choices and the actions you take to implement them are frequent concomitants of your decision to value your aliveness and the enjoyments that may go with it. But all these values and their derivatives not only are given to you (by your heredity and your environment) but also *accepted* and *chosen*. They are "good" because you (consciously or unconsciously) *decide* that they are. And even when you think that outside forces foist them on you or devoutly believe that God loves you (and that he or she *makes* you "good" or "worthwhile"), you obviously *choose* to believe this and thereby *select* the criteria for your human worth. If you are wise, therefore, you will admit that you make this choice and will consciously and honestly (from here on in) continue to make it.

To return to our central theme: If you insist on rating your *self* instead of merely rating your acts and traits, choose to see yourself as worthwhile simply because you exist. And try to see all other humans as "good" because they are human, because they are alive and have potential for enjoyments. If you, for purposes of your own, prefer to be with intelligent, cultured, tall, or any other kind of individuals, that is your privilege—go be with them. But if you insist that only intelligent, cultured, tall, or any other kind of individuals are good or worthy humans, you are, except by your personal and arbitrary definition, inaccurate, since you cannot present any unfalsifiable, scientific evidence to support your preference. Even if you induce the majority to agree with you—as, presumably, Mussolini, Hitler, and various other dictators have done—this merely proves that your view is popular, not that it is correct.

People, then, can be viewed as good in themselves—because they are people, because they exist. They may be good for some specific purpose because they have this or that trait. But that purpose *is* not them. Nor is this or that trait. If you want to use people for your purpose, then you can legitimately specify that they be intelligent, aesthethic, well educated, or what you will. But please don't, because you desire them to have certain traits, insist that they are worthless for not possessing these traits. Don't confuse their worthlessness to you with worthlessness in themselves.

This is the essence of intellectual fascism. It is a belief about humans that convinces not only the believers but usually their victims as well that people acquire intrinsic worth not from merely being, but from being intelligent, talented, competent, or achieving. It is politico-social fascism with the trait names changed—the same hearse with different license plates.

Appendix B
REBT Diminishes Much of the Human Ego

M uch of what we can call the human "ego" is vague and indeterminate and, when conceived of and given a global rating, interferes with survival and happiness. Certain aspects of ego seem to be vital and lead to beneficial results: for people do exist, or have aliveness, for a number of years, and they also have self-consciousness, or awareness of their existence. In this sense, they have uniqueness, ongoingness, and ego. What people call their "self" or "totality" or "personality," on the other hand, has a vague, almost indefinable quality. People may well have "good" or "bad" traits—characteristics that help or hinder them in their goals of survival or happiness—but they really have no *self* that *is* good or bad.

To increase their health and happiness, Rational Emotive Behavior Therapy (REBT) recommends that people had better resist the tendency to rate their *self* or *essence* and had better stick with only rating their deeds, traits, acts, characteristics, and performances. In some ways, they can also

Originally published by the Albert Ellis Institute, New York, 2002.

evaluate the *effectiveness* of how they think, feel, and do. Once they choose their goals and purposes, they can rate their efficacy and efficiency in achieving these goals. And as a number of experiments by Albert Bandura and his students have shown, their *belief* in their efficacy will often help make them more productive and achieving. But when people give a global, allover rating to their self or ego, they almost always create self-defeating, neurotic thoughts, feelings, and behaviors.

The vast majority of systems of psychotherapy seem intent on—indeed, almost obsessed with—upholding, bolstering, and strengthening people's "self-esteem." This includes such diverse systems as psychoanalysis, object relations, gestalt therapy, and even some of the main cognitive-behavior therapies. Very few systems of personality change, such as Zen Buddhism, take an opposing stand and try to help humans diminish or surrender some aspects of their egos, but these systems tend to have little popularity and to engender much dispute.

Carl Rogers ostensibly tried to help people achieve "unconditional positive regard" and thereby see themselves as "good persons" in spite of their lack of achievement. Actually, however, he induced them to regard themselves as "okay" through their having a good relationship with a psychotherapist. But that, unfortunately, makes their *self-*acceptance depend on their *therapist's* acting uncritically toward them. If so, that is still highly *conditional* acceptance, instead of the *un*conditional self-acceptance that REBT teaches.

REBT constitutes one of the few modern therapeutic schools that has taken something of a stand against ego-rating and continues to take an even stronger stand in this direction as it grows in its theory and its applications. This appendix outlines the up-to-date REBT position on ego-rating and explains why REBT helps people *diminish* their ego-rating propensities.

LEGITIMATE ASPECTS OF THE HUMAN EGO

REBT first tries to define the various aspects of the human ego and to endorse its "legitimate" aspects. It assumes that an individual's main goals or purposes include (1) remaining alive and healthy and (2) enjoying himself or herself—experiencing a good deal of happiness and relatively little pain or dissatisfaction. We may, of course, argue with these goals, and not everyone accepts them as "good." But assuming that a person does value them, then he or she may have a valid "ego," "self," "self-consciousness," or "personality" that we may conceive of as something along the following lines:

1. "I exist—have an ongoing aliveness that lasts many years and then apparently comes to an end, so that 'I' no longer exist."
2. "I exist separately, at least in part, from other humans, and can therefore conceive of myself as an individual in my 'own' right."

3. "I have different traits, at least in many of their details, from other humans, and consequently my 'I-ness' or my 'aliveness' has a certain kind of uniqueness. No other person in the entire world appears to have exactly the same traits as I have or equals 'me' or constitutes the same entity as 'me.'"

4. "I have the ability to keep existing, if I choose to do so, for a number of years—to have an ongoing existence and to have some degree of consistent traits as I continue to exist. In that sense, I remain 'me' for a long time, even though my traits change in important respects."

5. "I have awareness or consciousness of my ongoingness, of my existence, of my behaviors and traits, and of various other aspects of my aliveness and experiencing. I can therefore say, 'I have self-consciousness.'"

6. "I have some power to predict and plan for my future existence or ongoingness and to change some of my traits and behaviors in accordance with my basic values and goals. My 'rational behavior,' as Myles Friedman has pointed out, to a large extent consists of my ability to predict and plan for my future."

7. "Because of my 'self-consciousness' and my ability to predict and plan for the future, I can to a considerable degree change my present and future traits (and hence 'existence'). In other words, I can at least partially control 'myself.'"

8. "I similarly have the ability to remember, understand, and learn from my past and present experi-

ences and to use this remembering, understanding, and learning in the service of predicting and changing my future behavior."

9. "I can choose to discover what I like (enjoy) and dislike (disenjoy) and to try to arrange to experience more of what I like and less of what I dislike. I can also choose to survive or not to survive."

10. "I can choose to monitor or observe my thoughts, feelings, and actions to help myself survive and lead a more satisfying or more enjoyable existence."

11. "I can have confidence (believe that a high probability exists) that I can remain alive and make myself relatively happy and free from pain."

12. "I can choose to act as a *short-range* hedonist who mainly goes for the pleasures of the moment and gives little consideration to those of the future or as a *long-range* hedonist who considers both the pleasures of the moment and of the future and who strives to achieve a fair degree of both."

13. "I can choose to see myself as having worth or value for pragmatic reasons—because I will then tend to act in my own interests, to go for pleasures rather than pain, to survive better, and to feel good."

14. "I can choose to accept myself unconditionally—whether or not I do well or get approved by others. I can thereby refuse to rate 'myself', 'my totality', 'my personhood' at all. Instead, I can rate my traits, deeds, acts, and performances—for the purposes of surviving and enjoying my life more and *not* for the purposes of

'proving myself' *or* being 'egoistic' or showing that I have a 'better' or 'greater' value than others."

15. "My 'self' and my 'personality,' while in important ways individualistic and unique to me, are also very much part of my sociality and my culture. An unusually large part of "me" and how "I" think, feel, and behave is significantly influenced—and even created—by my social learning and my being involved in and influenced by various groups. I am far from being *merely* an individual in my *own* right. My personhood includes socialhood. Moreover, I rarely am a hermit but strongly *choose* to spend much of my life in family, school, work, neighborhood, community, and other *groups*. In numerous ways 'I' am 'me' and *also* a 'groupie'! 'My' individual ways of living, therefore, coalesce with 'social' rules of living. My 'self' is a personal *and* a social product—and process! My unconditional self-acceptance (USA) had better intrinsically include unconditional other-acceptance (UOA). I can—and will!—accept other people, as well as myself, with our virtues *and* our failings, with our important accomplishments *and* our nonachievements, just because we are alive and kicking, just because we are human! My survival and happiness are well worth striving for, and so are those of the rest of humanity."

These, it seems to me, are some "legitimate" aspects of ego-rating. Why legitimate? Because they seem to have some "reality"—that is, have some "facts" behind them. And because they appear to help people who subscribe to them to attain their usual basic chosen values of surviving and feeling happy rather than miserable.

SELF-DEFEATING ASPECTS
OF THE HUMAN "EGO" (SELF-RATING)

At the same time, people subscribe to some "illegitimate" aspects of the human "ego" or of self-rating, such as these:

1. "I exist not only as a unique person but as a *special* person. I am a *better individual* than other people because of my outstanding traits."
2. "I have a superhuman rather than merely a human quality. I can do things that other people cannot possibly do and deserve to be deified for doing these things."
3. "If I do not have outstanding, special, or super-human characteristics, I am subhuman. Whenever I do not perform notably, I deserve to be devil-ified and damned."
4. "The universe especially and signally cares about me. It has a personal interest in me and wants to see me do remarkably well and to feel happy."
5. "I *need* the universe to specially care about me. If it does not, I am a lowly individual, cannot take care of myself, and must feel desperately miserable."

6. "Because I exist, I *absolutely* have to succeed in life, and I *must* obtain love and approval from all the people whom I find significant."

7. "Because I exist, I *must* survive and *must* continue to have a happy existence."

8. "Because I exist, I *must* exist forever and have *immortality*."

9. "I *equal* my traits. If I have significant bad traits, *I* totally rate as bad, and if I have significant good ones, *I* rate as a good person."

10. "I particularly equal my character traits. If I treat others well and therefore have a 'good character,' I am a good person; if I treat others badly and therefore have a 'bad character,' I have the essence of a bad person."

11. "In order to accept and respect myself, I must prove I have real worth—prove it by having competence, outstandingness, and the approval of others."

12. "To have a happy existence, I *must* have—I absolutely *need*—the things I really want."

The self-rating aspects of ego, in other words, tend to do you in, to handicap you, to interfere with your satisfactions. They differ enormously from the self-individuating aspects of ego. The latter involve *how* or *how well* you exist. You remain alive as a distinct, different, and unique individual because you have various traits and performances and because you enjoy their fruits. But you have ego in the sense of self-rating because you magically think in terms of upping or downing, deifying or devilifying yourself *for* how or how well you exist. Ironically, you probably think that rating yourself or your "ego" will help you live as a unique person and enjoy yourself. Well, it usually won't! For the most part it will let you survive, perhaps—but pretty miserably!

ADVANTAGES OF "EGO-ISM" OR SELF-RATING

Doesn't "ego-ism", self-rating, or self-esteem have *any* advantages? It certainly does—and therefore, probably, it survives in spite of its disadvantages. What advantages does it have? It tends to motivate you to succeed and to win others' approval. It gives you an interesting, preoccupying *game* of constantly comparing your deeds and your *self* to those of other people. It often helps you impress others, which has a practical value, in many instances. It may help preserve your life—such as when you strive to make more money, for egoistic reasons, and thus aid your survival by means of this money.

Self-rating serves as a very easy and comfortable position to fall into—humans seem to have a biological tendency to engage in it. It can also give you enormous pleasure when you rate yourself as noble, great, or outstanding. It may motivate you to produce notable works of art, science, or invention. It can enable you to feel superior to others—at times, even to feel godlike.

Ego-ism obviously has real advantages. To give up self-rating completely would amount to quite a sacrifice. We cannot justifiably say that it brings no gains or produces no social or individual good.

DISADVANTAGES OF "EGO-ISM" OR SELF-RATING

These are some of the more important reasons why rating yourself as either a "good" or a "bad" person has immense dangers and will frequently handicap you:

1. To work well, self-rating requires you to have extraordinary ability and talent or virtual infallibility, for you then can only elevate your ego when you do well and concomitantly depress it when you do poorly. What chances do you have of consistently or always doing well?

2. To have, in common parlance, a "strong" ego or "real" self-esteem really requires you to be above average or outstanding. Only if you have special talent will you likely accept yourself and rate yourself highly. But, obviously, very few individuals can have unusual, geniuslike ability. And will you personally reach that uncommon level? I doubt it!

3. Even if you have enormous talents and abilities, to accept yourself or esteem yourself consistently, in an ego-rating way, you have to display them virtually all the time. Any significant lapse and you immediately tend to down yourself. And then, when you down yourself, you tend to lapse more—a truly vicious circle!

4. When you insist on gaining "self-esteem," you basically do so in order to impress others with your great "value" or "worth" as a human. But the need

to impress others and to win their approval, and thereby view yourself as a "good person," leads to an obsession that tends to preempt a large part of your life. You seek status instead of seeking joy. And you seek universal acceptance, which you certainly have virtually no chance of ever getting!

5. Even when you impress others, and supposedly gain "worth" that way, you tend to realize that you do so partly by acting and falsifying your talents. You consequently look upon yourself as a phony. Ironically, then, first you down yourself for not impressing others, but then you down yourself for phonily impressing them!

6. When you rate yourself and succeed at giving yourself a superior rating, you delude yourself into thinking you have superiority over others. You may indeed have some superior traits, but you devoutly feel that you become a truly superior person—or semigod. And that delusion gives you an artificial or false sense of "self-esteem."

7. When you insist on rating yourself as good or bad, you tend to focus on your defects, liabilities, and failings, for you feel certain that they make you into an R. P., or rotten person. By focusing on these defects, you accentuate them, often making them worse; interfere with changing them; and acquire a generalized negative view of yourself that frequently ends up in arrant self-deprecation.

8. When you rate your *self*, instead of evaluating only

the effectiveness of your thoughts, feelings, and actions, you have the philosophy that you *must* prove yourself as good, and since there always exists a good chance that you will not, you tend to remain underlyingly or overtly anxious practically all the time. In addition, you may continually verge on depression, despair, and feelings of intense shame, guilt, and worthlessness.

9. When you preoccupyingly rate yourself, even if you succeed in earning a good rating, you do so at the expense of becoming obsessed with success, achievement, attainment, and outstandingness. But this kind of concentration on success deflects you from doing what *you* really desire to do and from the goal of trying to be happy: Some of the most successful people actually remain quite miserable.

10. By the same token, in mightily striving for outstandingness, success, and superiority, you rarely stop to ask yourself, "What do I really want—and want for myself?" So you fail to find what you really enjoy in life.

11. Ostensibly, your focusing on achieving greatness and superiority over others and thereby winning a high self-rating serves to help you do better in life. Actually, it helps you focus on your so-called *worth* and *value* rather than on your competency and happiness; consequently, you fail to achieve many things that you otherwise could. Because you *have* to prove your utter competence, you often tend to

make yourself less competent—and sometimes withdraw from competition.

12. Although self-rating occasionally may help you pursue creative activities, it frequently has the opposite result. For example, you may become so hung up on success and superiority that you uncreatively and obsessively-compulsively go for those goals rather than that of creative participation in art, music, science, invention, or other pursuits.

13. When you rate yourself, you tend to become self-centered rather than problem-centered. Therefore, you do not try to solve many of the practical and important problems in life but largely focus on your own navel and the pseudoproblem of *proving* yourself instead of *finding* yourself.

14. Self-rating generally helps you feel abnormally self-conscious. Self-consciousness, or the knowledge that you have an ongoing quality and can enjoy or disenjoy yourself, can have great advantages. But extreme self-consciousness, or continually spying on yourself and rating yourself on how well you do, takes this good trait to an obnoxious extreme and may interfere seriously with your happiness.

15. Self-rating encourages a great amount of prejudice. It consists of an overgeneralization: "Because one or more of my traits seem inadequate, I rate as a totally inadequate person." This means, in effect, that you feel prejudiced against *yourself* for some of your *behavior*. In doing this, you tend also to feel preju-

diced against others for their poor behavior—or for what you consider their inferior traits. You thus can make yourself feel bigoted about blacks, Jews, Catholics, Italians, and various other groups that include some people you do not like.

16. Self-rating leads to necessitizing and compulsiveness. When you believe "I must down myself when I have a crummy trait or set of performances," you usually also believe that "I absolutely *have* to have good traits or performances," and you feel compelled to act in certain "good" ways—even when you have little chance of consistently doing so.

WHY "EGO-ISM" AND SELF-RATING ARE ILLOGICAL

In these and other ways, attempting to have "ego-strength" or "self-esteem" leads to distinctly poor results: meaning, it interferes with your life and happiness. To make matters even worse, ego-ratings or self-ratings are unsound, in that accurate or "true" self-ratings or global ratings are virtually impossible to make because a global or total rating of an individual involves the following kinds of contradictions and magical thinking:

1. As a person, you have almost innumerable traits—virtually all of which change from day to day or year to year. How can any single global rating of you, therefore, meaningfully apply to all of you—including

your constantly changing traits?

2. You exist as an ongoing *process*—an individual who has a past, present, and future. Any rating of your you-ness, therefore, would apply only to "you" at single points in time and hardly to your ongoingness.

3. To give a rating to "you" totally, we would have to rate all of your traits, deeds, acts, and performances and somehow add or multiply them. But these characteristics are valued differently in different cultures and at different times. And *who* can therefore legitimately rate or weight them, except in a given culture at a given time and to a very limited degree?

4. If we did get legitimate ratings for every one of your past, present, and future traits, what kind of math would we employ to total them? Can we divide by the number of traits and get a "valid" global rating? Could we use simple arithmetic? Algebraic ratings? Geometric ratings? Logarithmic ratings? What?

5. To rate "you" totally and accurately, we would have to know the "important" traits and include them in our total. But how could we ever know them all? All your thoughts? Your emotions? Your "good" and "bad" deeds? Your accomplishments? Your psychological state?

6. To say that you have no value or are worthless involves several unprovable (and unfalsifiable) hypotheses: (1) that you have, innately, an essence of worthlessness; (2) that you never could possibly have any worth whatsoever; and (3) that you deserve

damnation or eternal punishment for having the mis-
fortune or worthlessness. Similarly, to say that you
have great worth involves the unprovable hypothesis
that (1) you just happen to have superior worth; (2)
you will always have it, no matter what you do; and
(3) you deserve deification or eternal reward for
having this boon of great worth. No scientific
methods of confirming or falsifying these hypotheses
seem to exist.

7. When you posit global worth or worthlessness, you
almost inevitably get yourself into circular thinking.
If you *see* yourself as having intrinsic value, you will
tend to *see* your traits as good and will have a halo
effect. Then you will falsely conclude that because
you have these good characteristics, you have intrinsic
value. Similarly, if you see yourself as having worthlessness, you will view your "good" traits as "bad"
and "prove" your hypothesized lack of value.

8. You can pragmatically believe that "I am good because
I exist." But this stands as a tautological, unprovable
hypothesis, in the same class with the equally unprovable (and undisprovable) statement, "I am bad
because I exist." *Assuming* that you have intrinsic value
because you remain alive may help you feel happier
than if you assume the opposite. But philosophically,
it remains an untenable proposition. You might just
as well say, "I have worth because God loves me," or "I
have no value because God (or the Devil) hates me."
The assumptions cause you to feel and act in certain

ways, but they appear essentially unverifiable and unfalsifiable.

For reasons such as those just outlined, we may make the following conclusions: (1) You do seem to exist, or have aliveness, for a number of years, and you also appear to have consciousness, or awareness of your existence. In this sense, you have a human uniqueness, ongoingness, or, if you will, "ego." (2) But what you normally call your "self" or your "totality" or your "personality" has a vague, almost indefinable quality, and you cannot legitimately give it a global rating or report card. You may *have* good and bad traits or characteristics that help you or hinder you in your goals of survival and happiness and that enable you to live responsibly or irresponsibly with others. But you or your "self" really "aren't" good or bad. (3) When you give yourself a global rating, or have "ego" in the usual sense of that term, you may help yourself in various ways; on the whole, however, you tend to do much more harm than good and preoccupy yourself with rather foolish, side-tracking goals. Much of what we call emotional "disturbance" or neurotic "symptoms" directly or indirectly results from globally rating yourself and other humans. (4) Therefore, you'd better resist the tendency to rate your *self* or your *essence* or your *totality* and had better stick with only rating your deeds, traits, acts, characteristics, and performances.

In other words, you had better reduce much of what we normally call your human "ego" and retain those parts of it that can help you experiment with life, choose what you tentatively think you want to do or avoid, and enjoy what you *discover* is "good" for you and for the social group in which you choose to live.

More positively, the two main solutions to the problem of self-rating consist of an inelegant and an elegant answer. The inelegant solution involves your making an arbitrary but practical definition or statement about yourself: "I accept myself as good or evaluate myself as good because I exist." This proposition, though arguable, will tend to provide you with feelings of self-acceptance or self-confidence and has many advantages and few disadvantages. It will almost always work and will preclude your having feelings of self-denigration or worthlessness as long as you hold it.

More elegantly, you can accept this proposition: "I do not have intrinsic worth or worthlessness but merely aliveness. I'd better rate my traits and acts but not my totality or 'self.' I fully *accept* myself, in the sense that I know I have aliveness, and I *choose* to survive and live as happily as possible, and with minimum needless pain. I only require this knowledge and this choice—and no other kind of self-rating."

In other words, you can decide to rate or measure only your *acts* and *performances*—your thoughts, feelings, and behaviors—by viewing them as "good" when they aid your goals and values and as "bad" when they sabotage your individual and social desires and preferences. But you can simultaneously decide not to rate your *self*, *essence*, or *totality* at all. Yes, *at all*!

Rational Emotive Behavior Therapy (REBT) recommends this second, more elegant solution, because it appears more honest and more practical and leads to fewer philosophical difficulties than the inelegant one. But if you absolutely insist on a self-rating, we recommend that you rate yourself as "good" *merely* because you are alive. That kind of "ego-ism" will get you into very little trouble!

Selected References

The following references include the works of the main authors mentioned in this book—but by no means all of them. A good many of these authors are famous writers and philosophers whose standard works can be found in most bookstores and libraries. An additional number of publications on Rational Emotive Behavior Therapy (REBT) and Cognitive Behavior Therapy (CBT) have been included because they are useful for understanding the theory and practice of REBT and CBT and for self-help purposes. Many of the references may be obtained from the Albert Ellis Institute, 45 East 65th Street, New York, NY 10021. The Institute's free catalog includes many books, cassettes, and live presentations on psychotherapy, which may be ordered by phone ([212] 535-0822), by mail (45 East 65th Street New York, NY 10021), by fax ([212] 249-3582), or by e-mail (orders@rebt.org). The Institute will continue to make available talks, workshops, and training sessions as well as other presentations in the area of human growth and health and will list these in its regular catalog and on its Web site (http://www.rebt.org).

Selected References

Adler, A. *The Science of Living*. New York: Greenberg, 1929.

Ansbacher, H. L., and R. Ansbacher. *The Individual Psychology of Alfred Adler*. New York: Basic Books, 1956.

Bandura, A. *Self-Efficacy: The Exercise of Control*. New York: Freeman, 1997.

Barlow, D. H., and N. G. Craske. *Mastery of Your Anxiety and Panic*. Albany: Graywind Publications, 1994.

Beck, A. T. *Cognitive Therapy and the Emotional Disorders*. New York: International Universities Press, 1976.

———. *Love Is Not Enough*. New York: Harper & Row, 1988.

Beck, A. T., A. J. Rush, B. F. Shaw, and G. Emery. *Cognitive Therapy of Depression*. New York: Guilford, 1979.

Bernard, M. E. *Staying Rational in an Irrational World*. New York: Citadel Press, 1993.

Bernard, M. E., and A. Ellis. "Albert Ellis at 85: Professional Reflections." *Journal of Rational-Emotive and Cognitive-Behavior Therapy* 16 (1998): 151–81.

———. "Albert Ellis at 85: Personal Reflections." *Journal of Rational-Emotive and Cognitive Behavior Therapy* 16 (1998): 213–22.

Bernard, M. E., and J. L. Wolfe, eds. *The REBT Resource Book for Practitioners*. New York: Albert Ellis Institute, 2000.

Bishop, M. *Managing Addictions: Cognitive and Behavioral Techniques*. Holmes, PA: Aaronson, 2001.

Bowlby, J. *Attachment and Loss*, vol. 1: *Attachment*. New York: Basic Books, 1969.

Branden, N. *Judgment Day: My Years with Ayn Rand*. Boston: Houghton Mifflin, 1989.

Broder, M. S. *The Art of Living*. New York: Avon, 1990.

Buber, M. *I and Thou*. New York: Scribner, 1984.

Burns, D. D. *Feeling Good: The New Mood Therapy*. Rev. ed. New York: William Morrow, 1999.

Cohen, Elliot D. *What Would Aristotle Do? Self-Control through the Power of Reason.* Amherst, NY: Prometheus Books, 2003.

Crawford, T., and A. Ellis. "A Dictionary of Rational-Emotive Feelings and Behaviors." *Journal of Rational-Emotive and Cognitive-Behavior Therapy* 7, no. 1 (1989): 3–27.

Dewey, J. *Quest for Certainty.* New York: Putnam, 1929.

DiGiuseppe, R. "The Implication of the Philosophy of Science for Rational-Emotive Theory and Therapy." *Psychotherapy* 23 (1986): 634–39.

DiGiuseppe, R., M. Robin, and W. Dryden. "On the Compatibility of RET and Judeo-Christian Philosophy." *Journal of Cognitive Therapy* 4, no. 4 (1990): 355–67.

DiMattia, D., and L. Lega, eds. *Will the Real Albert Ellis Please Stand Up? Anecdotes by His Colleagues, Students, and Friends Celebrating His 75th Birthday.* New York: Albert Ellis Institute, 1990.

Dryden, W. *Brief Rational Emotive Behavior Therapy.* London: Wiley, 1995.

———. *How to Accept Yourself.* London: Sheldon, 1999.

———. *Reason to Change: A Rational Emotive Behavior Therapy (REBT) Workbook.* Hove, England: Brunner-Routledge, 2001.

Dryden, W., R. DiGiuseppe, and M. Neenan. *A Primer on Rational-Emotive Therapy.* Champaign, IL: Research Press, 2003.

Dryden, W., and A. Ellis. *Albert Ellis Live.* London: Sage, 2003.

Dryden, W., and J. Gordon. *Think Your Way to Happiness.* London: Sheldon, 1991.

Dryden, W., and M. Neenan. *The Rational Emotive Behavioral Approach to Therapeutic Change.* London: Sage, 2003.

Dryden, W., J. Walker, and A. Ellis. *REBT Self-Help Form.* New York: Albert Ellis Institute, 1996.

Edelstein, M., and D. R. Steele. *Three-Minute Therapy: Change Your Life.* Lakewood, CO: Glenbridge, 1997.

Selected References

Ellis, A. *The Art and Science of Love*. New York: Lyle Stuart & Bantam, 1960.

———. *The American Sexual Tragedy*. Rev. ed. New York: Lyle Stuart and Grove Press, 1962.

———. *Reason and Emotion in Psychotherapy*. Secaucus, NJ: Citadel, 1962.

———. *Is Objectivism a Religion?* New York: Lyle Stuart, 1968.

———. *Psychotherapy and the Value of a Human Being*. New York: Albert Ellis Institute, 1972.

———. "The Biological Basis of Human Irrationality." *Journal of Individual Psychology* 32 (1976): 145–68.

———. *The Case against Religiosity*. New York: Albert Ellis Institute, 1983.

———. "Fanaticism That May Lead to a Nuclear Holocaust: The Contributions of Scientific Counseling and Psychotherapy." *Journal of Counseling and Development* 65 (1986): 146–51.

———. *How to Stubbornly Refuse to Make Yourself Miserable about Anything—Yes, Anything!* New York: Kensington Publishers, 1988.

———. *Unconditionally Accepting Yourself and Others*. Cassette recording. New York: Albert Ellis Institute, 1992.

——— *Reason and Emotion in Psychotherapy*. Rev. and upd. ed. New York: Kensington Publishers, 1994.

———. *How to Maintain and Enhance Your Rational Emotive Behavior Therapy Gains*. Rev. ed. New York: Albert Ellis Institute, 1996.

———. *How to Make Yourself Happy and Remarkably Less Disturbable*. Atascadero, CA: Impact Publishers, 1999.

———. *My Philosophy of Psychotherapy*. Rev. ed. New York: Institute for Rational Emotive Behavior Therapy, 1996.

———. *How to Control Your Anxiety before It Controls You*. New York: Citadel, 2000.

————. *How to Maintain and Enhance Your Rational Emotive Therapy Gains.* New York: Albert Ellis Institute, 2000.

————. *Feeling Better, Getting Better, and Staying Better.* Atascadero, CA: Impact Publishers, 2001.

————. *Overcoming Destructive Beliefs, Feelings, and Behaviors.* Amherst, NY: Prometheus Books, 2001.

————. *Overcoming Resistance: A Rational Emotive Behavior Therapy Integrative Approach.* New York: Springer, 2002.

————. *Anger: How to Live with and without It.* Rev. ed. New York: Citadel, 2003.

————. *Ask Albert Ellis.* Atascadero, CA: Impact Publishers, 2003.

————. *Sex without Guilt for the Twenty-first Century.* Teaneck, NJ: Barricade, 2003.

————. *Rational Emotive Behavior Therapy: It Works for Me—It Can Work for You.* Amherst, NY: Prometheus Books, 2004.

Ellis, A., and S. Blau, eds. *The Albert Ellis Reader.* New York: Citadel Books, 1997.

Ellis, A., and T. Crawford. *Making Intimate Connections: Seven Guidelines for Great Relationships and Better Communication.* Atascadero, CA: Impact Publishers, 2000.

Ellis, A., and W. Dryden. *The Practice of Rational Emotive Behavior Therapy.* New York: Springer, 1997.

Ellis, A., V. Gordon, M. Neenan, and S. Palmer. *Stress Counseling.* New York: Springer, 1998.

Ellis, A., and R. A. Harper. *A Guide to Rational Living.* Rev. ed. North Hollywood, CA: Melvin Powers Wilshire Books, 1961. Reprint, 1977.

————. *Dating, Mating, and Relating: How to Build a Healthy Relationship.* New York: Citadel, 2002.

Ellis, A., and W. Knaus. *Overcoming Procrastination.* New York: New American Library, 1977.

| Selected References

Ellis, A., and A. Lange. *How to Keep People from Pushing Your Buttons.* New York: Citadel, 2003.

Ellis, A., and C. MacLaren. *Rational Emotive Behavior Therapy: A Therapist's Guide.* Atascadero, CA: Impact Publishers, 1998.

Ellis, A., J. L. Sichel, R. J. Yeager, D. J. DiMattia, and R. A. DiGiuseppe. *Rational-Emotive Couples Therapy.* Needham, MA: Allyn & Bacon, 1989.

Ellis, A., and C. Tafrate. *How to Control Your Anger before It Controls You.* New York: Citadel, 1998.

Ellis, A., and E. Velten. *When AA Doesn't Work for You: Rational Steps for Quitting Alcohol.* New York: Barricade Books, 1992.

———. *Optimal Aging: Getting Over Getting Older.* Chicago: Open Court, 1998.

Ellis. A., and J. M. Whiteley. *Theoretical and Empirical Foundations of Rational-Emotive Therapy.* Monterey, CA: Brooks/Cole, 1979.

Ellis, A., J. L. Wolfe, and S. Mosley. *How to Raise an Emotionally Healthy, Happy Child.* North Hollywood, CA: Wilshire Books, 1966.

FitzMaurice, K. E. *Attitude Is All You Need.* Omaha: Palm Tree Publishers, 1997.

Freud, S. *Basic Writings.* New York: Modern Library, 1938.

Kelly, G. *The Psychology of Personal Constructs.* New York: Norton, 1955.

Kemmler, L. *"Wandelt euch duce en neves denken." Ein Vergleich von zwei Begriffen der RET und vinegen Aussagen jesus von nazgus in neven testament. Zutschuft fur rational emotive & kugnitive verhaltens therapie* 11 (2000): 1–34.

Kirsch, I. *How Expectations Shape Experience.* Washington, DC: American Psychological Association, 1999.

Korzybski, A. *Science and Sanity.* Concord, CA: International Society for General Semantics, 1933. Reprint, 1990.

Kurtz, P. *The Transcendental Temptation.* Amherst, NY: Prometheus Books, 1986.

Kwee, M. G. T., and A. Ellis. "Can Multimodal and Rational Emotive Behavior Therapy Be Reconciled?" *Journal of Rational-Emotive and Cognitive-Behavior Therapy* 15, no. 2 (1997): 95–132.

Lao-Tsu. *Tao: A New Way of Thinking.* New York: Harper & Row, 1975.

Lazarus, A. A. *The Practice of Multimodal Therapy.* Baltimore: Johns Hopkins University Press, 1989.

Lazarus, R. S. *Stress and Emotion: A New Synthesis.* New York: Springer, 1999.

Low, A. A. *Mental Health through Will Training.* Boston: Christopher, 1952.

Lyons, L. C., and P. J. Woods. "The Efficacy of Rational Emotive Therapy: A Quantative Review of the Outcome Research." *Clinical Psychology Review* 11 (1991): 357–69.

Mahoney, M. J. *Human Change Processes.* New York: Basic Books, 1991.

Masters, W. H., and V. E. Johnson. *Human Sexual Response.* Boston: Houghton Mifflin, 1960.

Maultsby, M. C., Jr. "Rational Emotive Imagery." *Rational Living* 6, no. 1 (1971): 16–23.

———. *Rational Behavior Therapy.* Englewood Cliffs, NJ: Prentice-Hall, 1984.

McGinn, L. K. "Interview with Albert Ellis." *American Journal of Psychotherapy* 51 (1997): 309–16.

Meichenbaum, D. "The Evolution of a Cognitive Behavior Therapist." In *The Evolution of Psychotherapy: The Third Conference,* edited by J. K. Zeig. New York: Brunner/Mazel, 1997, pp. 95–106.

Pillay, A. P., and A. Ellis, eds. *Sex, Society, and the Individual.* Bombay: International Journal of Sexology, 1953.

Rogers, C. R. *On Becoming a Person.* Boston: Houghton Mifflin, 1961.

Reiss, I. L., and A. Ellis. *At the Dawn of the Sexual Revolution.* Walnut Creek, CA: Altamira Press, 2002.

Robb, H. B. "Facilitating REBT by Including Religious Beliefs." *Cognition and Behavioral Practice* 8 (2001): 29–34.

Russell, B. *Marriage and Morals*. New York: Simon & Schuster, 1929.

Suzuki, D. T., E. Fromm, and R. De Martino. *Zen Buddhism and Psychoanalysis*. New York: Harper, 1960.

Tillich, P. *The Courage to Be*. Cambridge: Harvard University Press, 1953.

Walen, S., R. DiGiuseppe, and W. Dryden. *A Practitioner's Guide to Rational-Emotive Therapy*. New York: Oxford University Press, 1992.

Watts, A. W. *Nature, Man, and Woman*. New York: New American Library, 1958.

Watzlawick, P. *The Language of Change*. New York: Basic Books, 1978.

Wiener, D. *Albert Ellis: Passionate Skeptic*. New York: Praeger, 1988.

Weinrach, S. G. "Rational Emotive Behavior Therapy: A Tough-Minded Therapy for a Tender-Minded Profession." *Journal of Counseling and Development* 73 (1995): 296–300. Reprinted in *Rational Emotive Behavior Therapy: A Reader*, edited by W. Dryden. London: Sage, 1995, pp. 303–12.

Wolfe, J. L. *What to Do When He Has a Headache*. New York: Hyperion, 1992.

Woods, P. J. *Controlling Your Smoking: A Comprehensive Set of Strategies for Smoking Reduction*. Roanoke, VA: Scholars Press, 1990.

Young, H. S. *A Rational Counseling Primer*. New York: Albert Ellis Institute, 1974.

About the Author

Albert Ellis was born in Pittsburgh and raised in New York City. He holds MA and PhD degrees in clinical psychology from Columbia University. He has held many important psychological positions, including chief psychologist of the state of New Jersey and adjunct professorships at Rutgers and other universities. He is currently president of the Albert Ellis Institute in New York City; has practiced psychotherapy, marriage and family counseling, and sex therapy for sixty years; and continues this practice at the Psychological Center of the institute in New York. He is the founder of Rational Emotive Behavior Therapy (REBT), the first of the now-popular Cognitive Behavior Therapies (CBT).

Dr. Ellis has served as president of the Division of Consulting Psychology of the American Psychological Association and of the Society for the Scientific Study of Sexuality, and he has also served as officer of several professional societies, including the American Association of Marital and Family Therapy; the American Academy of Psychotherapists; and the American Academy of Sex Educators, Counselors, and Therapists. He is a diplomat in clinical psychology of the American Board of Professional Psychology and of several other professional organizations.

Professional societies that have given Dr. Ellis their highest professional and clinical awards include the American Psychological Association, the Association for the Advancement of Behavior Therapy, the American Counseling Association, and the American Psychopathological Association. He was ranked as one of the "most influential psychologists" by both the American and Canadian psychologists and counselors. He has served as consulting or associate editor of many scientific journals and has published over eight hundred scientific papers and more than two hundred audio- and videocassettes. He has written or edited seventy-five books and monographs, including a number of best-selling popular and professional volumes. Some of his best-known books include *How to Live with a "Neurotic"*; *The Art and Science of Love*; *A Guide to Rational Living*; *Reason and Emotion in Psychotherapy*; *How to Stubbornly Refuse to Make Yourself Miserable about Anything—Yes, Anything*; *Overcoming Procrastination*; *Overcoming Resistance*; *The Practice of Rational Emotive Behavior Therapy*; *How to Make Yourself Happy and Remarkably Less Disturbable*; *Feeling Better, Getting Better, and Staying Better*; *Overcoming Destructive Beliefs, Feelings, and Behaviors*; *Anger: How to Live with It and without It*; and *Rational Emotive Behavior Therapy: It Works for Me—It Can Work for You*.

Index

AA. *See* Alcoholics Anonymous

Aaron's Rod (Lawrence), 57–58

A-B-C of rational psychotherapy, 32–36, 80–81

abreaction, 46–48

absolutism, 13, 26–27, 113

achieving major goals and purposes, comparison of REBT and religious views, 122–23

activity lauding vs. self-lauding, 93

See also self-rating

Adler, Alfred, 44–45, 163, 169, 178, 195

Adlerian school of therapy, 44–45, 48

adolescents. *See* teenagers

adversity, 80

Albert Ellis Institute (New York City), 41–42, 84, 89, 184

Alcoholics Anonymous, 27, 205–206

altruism, 55–56

American Academy of Psychotherapists, 195

American Counseling Association, 84

American Journal of Psychotherapy, 78

American Psychological Association, 25, 84

The American Sexual Tragedy (Ellis), 176

Anger: How to Live with It and without It (Ellis), 88

antiawfulizing methods, 94, 96

See also awfulizing experiences

antiempiricism, 100–104

See also empiricism

antiextremism, 25–28

antimasturbation, 58–60

antimusturbatory philosophies, 24–25

See also musturbation